Ove

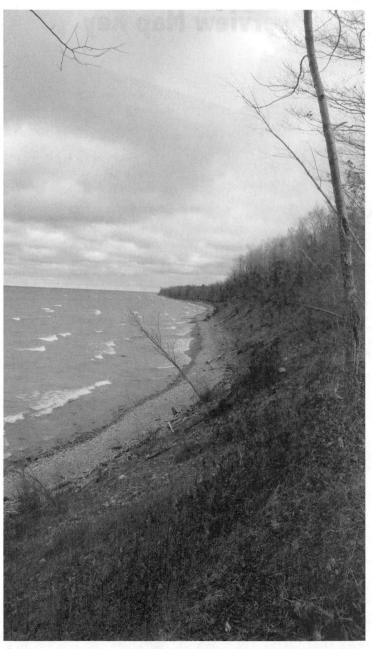

TRAIL 1 SHORE OF LAKE ONTARIO AT STERLING NATURE CENTER *see page 30*

Five-Star Trails

Finger Lakes
& Central New York

Your Guide to the Area's Most Beautiful Hikes

Timothy Starmer

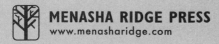
MENASHA RIDGE PRESS
www.menasharidge.com

Dedication

To my parents, who fostered a love of the outdoors in me. And also to Jake, Will, and Hannah in hopes that it inspires them with a similar love of the outdoors.

Five-Star Trails Finger Lakes & Central New York
Your Guide to the Area's Most Beautiful Hikes

Copyright © 2014 by Timothy Starmer
All rights reserved
Printed in the United States of America
Published by Menasha Ridge Press
Distributed by Publishers Group West
First edition, third printing 2022

Library of Congress Cataloging-in-Publication Data

Starmer, Timothy, 1975-
  Five-star trails, Finger Lakes and Central New York : your guide to the area's most beautiful hikes / Timothy Starmer.
    pages cm
  ISBN 978-0-89732-996-5 (paperback) — ISBN 0-89732-996-1
  1. Hiking—New York (State)—Finger Lakes region—Guidebooks. 2. Finger Lakes Region (N.Y.)—Guidebooks. I. Title.
  GV199.42.N652
  796.5109747—dc23
                         2014028500

Cover design by Scott McGrew
Text design by Annie Long
All interior and cover photographs by Timothy Starmer
Cartography and elevation profiles by Scott McGrew and Timothy Starmer

Menasha Ridge Press
An imprint of AdventureKEEN
2204 First Avenue South, Suite 102
Birmingham, Alabama 35233
menasharidge.com

DISCLAIMER

This book is meant only as a guide to select trails in and near the Finger Lakes area and Central New York. This book does not guarantee hiker safety in any way—you hike at your own risk. Neither Menasha Ridge Press nor Timothy Starmer is liable for property loss or damage, personal injury, or death that result in any way from accessing or hiking the trails described in the following pages. Please be especially cautious when walking in potentially hazardous terrains with, for example, steep inclines or drop-offs. Do not attempt to explore terrain that may be beyond your abilities. Please read carefully the introduction to this book, as well as further safety information from other sources. Familiarize yourself with current weather reports and maps of the area you plan to visit (in addition to the maps provided in this guidebook). Know park regulations, and always follow them. Do not take chances.

Contents

West 230

Appendixes 275

Acknowledgments

FIRST, I WOULD LIKE TO THANK EVERYONE at Menasha Ridge Press for allowing me once again to write about my hobby and passion. It's a privilege to do so. Maybe more important, I thank them for the patience and understanding that work on this book had to come second to my primary business.

Second, I must thank my parents for reading my drafts and helping in innumerable ways to make this possible.

Finally, I want to acknowledge the tireless efforts of the trail crews, volunteers, and professionals who build and maintain the trails. Your work is greatly admired and appreciated.

—*Timothy Starmer*

Preface

I SET OUT WRITING THIS BOOK because I enjoyed working on my first hiking book, *Five-Star Trails in the Adirondacks*. Part of me really wanted to go back to hike more of those wild and rugged trails and write part two. But also nagging at me was the desire to explore more in my own backyard, the Finger Lakes and Central New York regions. So when I approached the editors at Menasha Ridge Press about writing a second book, I presented both options. Obviously they chose the second, but at the outset I still held on to the idea that this book and its trails would be much like my first. I could not have been more wrong.

There are few soaring vistas, no mountains, and few boundless wilderness areas. Those are the trails I normally love and am drawn to. No, the trails here are not rugged and wild Adirondack trails, but they are not desert trails or rain forest trails either. They are what the region is: trails along drumlins, lakeside strolls, ascents of steeply sided hills and descents through U-shaped valleys, routes to staggeringly beautiful waterfalls, paths through scenic gorges, and hikes in quiet woodlands.

Many of the trails are found in state and county parks and include a level of development that is not typically associated with "hiking" trails. But there is a reason these parks were established and chosen. Within these parks are some astonishing gems of nature well worth visiting for even the most reclusive and hard-core hiker. As is the case with most parks and natural wonders, solitude here is rare, but I managed to find a few preserves and state forests for those who desire seclusion and wilderness.

Furthermore, the trails in the region pose relatively few physical challenges. In the Adirondacks a 3-mile hike can prove exhausting as you scramble up nearly vertical ascents and navigate bone-jarring descents, and several hours are often required for trips of even modest length. Here, the trails are mostly level and a motivated hiker can

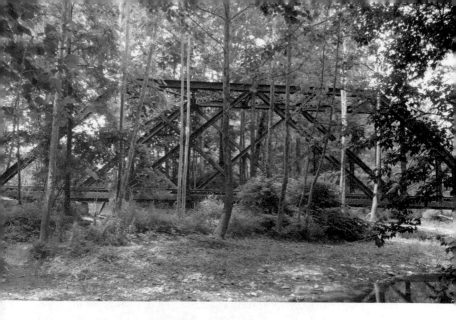

TRAIL 24 RAILROAD BRIDGE AT SWEEDLER PRESERVE *see page 182*

speedily cover ground at near running speeds. It was common for me to clock 4 or 5 miles an hour along the trails, far faster than the standard 2–3 miles an hour normally used as a baseline for planning a trip. As an aside, I still recommend using the 2- to 3-mile-per-hour metric for planning.

As I began my research, I soon realized there was little in the way of resources for the few trails that are scattered over this sprawling region. The descriptions I found were brief, and practically none explained what to expect along the trail. Cursory glances at chosen routes often led me to surprising encounters. Along one trail, I unexpectedly passed within feet of a sewage plant, and along many others I found myself trudging on roads more than trails. Don't worry; I have omitted these trails for obvious reasons. Initially, the maps I found for the trails were either useless or poorly illustrative of what to expect. The maps provided within this book should rectify these omissions, but I also strongly recommend the excellent maps provided by the Finger Lakes Trail Conference.

In the end this is not the book I set out to write, but as I researched and hiked the trails, it became one I know is necessary.

And as the research and hikes progressed, the region won me over with its marvels and the deeper story it holds within. There is more to this landscape than meets the eye. Whereas the Adirondack region is a narrative of wilderness—both by its nature and its preservation—the primary tale here is one of water and ice.

Ancient in genesis and long in evolving, the landscape today is a primeval seabed, uplifted, slowly eroded, and then dramatically carved and scoured by miles-thick sheets of ice. Where possible, I have tried to weave the history of the landscape with the trail descriptions, though the story shared in these pages is only partially told; its full telling is found by exploring, seeing, and experiencing the landscape in its own right. But the tale of water and ice is the common thread among the trails since they have no common forest, park, boundary, or agency. Indeed even the organization of the trails into regions is somewhat arbitrary. But consistent through all is a landscape shaped by water and ice. Glacial carved lakes, lakes formed as plunge pools at the base of miles-high sheets of ice, hanging valleys and waterfalls, innumerable fossils, gullies, gorges in their infancy, gorges that have been cut into canyons, drumlins, kettles, kames, ancient moraines, overly steepened wooded hilltops with odd U-shaped valleys in between—all created by water and ice. Looking at the trails through this lens, you may find them more intriguing and also discover a deeper connection to the region. But more on this landscape of water and ice later.

Recommended Hikes

Best for Fall Color

Best Geology

Best for Gorges

Best for Kids

Best for Lakes

Best for Seclusion

Best for Vistas

Best for Waterfalls

Best for Wildlife

Introduction

About This Book

I SELECTED TRAILS that give the broadest range of experiences to the broadest range of hikers and that illustrate a region's deeper story. Daylong rigorous treks are great for the diehard, experienced hikers but are a poor choice for novices and kids. So a hike may be a five-star trail because it would be great for a family with children, but crowds or lack of difficulty might eschew the seasoned backpacker. Other featured hikes are worth dealing with crowds to see the natural wonders. Some were chosen simply because solitude was virtually guaranteed, or they offer a bit more of a rigorous challenge, even though no great vistas or waterscapes are present.

To assist you in choosing which trail might best match your hiking style, a rating system has been used (see "Star Ratings," page 8). Also included are "Recommended Hikes," on pages xi–xii, so you can quickly find a trail that has characteristics best suited to your taste. Elevation profiles, included with hikes that have significant elevation change, illustrate the degree of climbing and difficulty you will experience on a trip (see "Elevation Profile," page 7). I encourage you to check out all the trails, even if you typically prefer one type over another, because taken as a whole, they offer unique perspectives on what help shaped this landscape and what makes the region unique.

Natural History & the Deeper Story Behind the Trails

There are no mountains in Central New York or the Finger Lakes area. Rather the region is dotted with hills, practically equal in height, and bisected by broad U-shaped valleys. Sometimes these valleys are filled with long sinuous lakes, two of which extend deep below sea level, an oddity that should alert you that something peculiar is going on with their formation. In others, the broad valley floors are bereft of a river or stream that could account for their shape or breadth. If you grew up in Central New York like I did, this may seem the natural way of things, but if you hike or travel in other parts of the world, you soon realize that there is something different about this landscape. This unusual topography is the result of multiple phases of land-forming processes, and in many ways it ties the trails described in this book together.

The first phase is evident whenever you explore a streambed or examine the stratified layers of rock along the dramatic gorge walls and stone amphitheaters that enclose the area's stunning waterfalls. What you see is layer upon layer of rock formed when New York was a part of a great inland sea. Embedded within are the fossilized remains of primeval sea life that reveal the truly ancient genesis of this landscape. The process took hundreds of millions of years as continents, bearing little resemblance to what we see today, collided. Mountains neighboring the inland sea were uplifted and then eroded away over eons, forming uniform layers of sandstone, shale, and limestone. After the staggering collision and union of continents into the single continent of Pangaea, plate tectonics shifted again, the continents began to separate, and a process of stretching and uplift began. Eventually the inland sea filled in and evaporated, creating the wide salt beds that Syracuse is founded around and renowned for. The once-level seabed was tilted upward, but then the Northeast underwent a period of relative geologic stability. Far from the leading edge of plate tectonic activity occurring out in the widening Atlantic Ocean, the landscape "settled down," millennia of slow erosion broke down soft layers and left harder erosion-resistant layers, and the basic shape of the modern landscape emerged. Here the story takes a turn and something dramatic occurs that sets this topography apart. What took shape over hundreds of millions of years in a slow process was drastically and rapidly altered by advancing sheets of miles-deep ice.

The tale now shifts to the transformative power of glaciers, the irony being that the glacial process—a term we often associate with being slow—was a surprisingly rapid transformation, respective to geological time, of course. During the ice age known as the Pleistocene epoch, the advance of the ice was swift—several feet per day. Even today that would be remarkable, especially when you consider that the ice we are talking about was continental in scale and miles thick. The ice sheet was so massive that not only did it depress the landscape far below its present-day elevation, but the land is also still rebounding from the glacier's departure. Perhaps even more astonishing is that it continues to rebound at a rate that is predicted, albeit far in the future, to reverse the flow of Niagara Falls.

The epoch started around 1.8 million years ago and ended only 10,000 years ago, a relatively short time frame when compared to the hundreds of millions of years that preceded it. Virtually no area in New York remained untouched by the glaciers (the Salamanca Reentrant in Allegany State Park is the only exception). Temperatures were at least 5° colder worldwide. Central New Yorkers are no strangers to long winters and feet of snow lasting for months, but during the Pleistocene snow remained year-round and extended as far south as New Jersey. The snow accumulated faster than it melted, and the massive ice sheets eventually fell into a self-propagating system. The larger the ice sheets became, the more sun they reflected, cooling the environment and leading to more snowfall and less melting. Glaciers were becoming continental forces. One-third of the Earth's land surface was covered by ice.

Originating around the Hudson Bay area of Canada, the massive Laurentide sheet of ice advanced and retreated multiple times, each time scouring and depositing staggering amounts of glacial till. In New York, evidence of earlier advances was mostly scrubbed clean by the most recent phase: the Wisconsinan Stage, in which the processes that shaped our current landscape took place. River valleys were gouged ever deeper. The bottoms of Seneca and Cayuga Lakes are actually 173 and 51 feet below sea level respectively. As the glacier retreated, it left behind staggering amounts of material along its leading edge, forming moraines that run perpendicular to its flow. When the advance or recession of the ice stalled in one place, the moraines became immense. If you consider that Long Island is essentially one large glacial deposit, then you begin to grasp the scale of a continental-size bulldozer.

In the Finger Lakes region, an immense moraine, the Valley Heads Moraine, is believed to have formed over a 200- to 500-year period when the supply and melting of ice was in a state of equilibrium. The Valley Head dammed rivers that once flowed south into the Susquehanna watershed in Pennsylvania. In the area, the direction in which streams flow is often indicative of this divide. For example, the Texas Hollow stream, page 170, and Cayuta Creek in the Connecticut Hill Wildlife Management Area, page 209, are roughly 5 miles apart. But the former flows north and eventually into the Saint Lawrence River Valley, while the latter flows south into the Susquehanna and on to the Chesapeake Bay.

With nowhere for meltwater to flow, immense lakes formed between the moraine and receding ice sheet. These glacial lake levels were much higher than today. As the ice slowly retreated north, the levels would drop, creating hanging valleys, and streams that once emptied directly into lakes now cascaded in dramatic waterfalls. Taughannock Falls, pages 133 and 139, is the most stunning example of this phenomenon, but all of the region's gorges were formed in a similar fashion.

Elsewhere where the ice stalled, great waterfalls gouged out deep plunge pools to form deep pothole lakes; Glacier Lake at Clark Reservation State Park, page 70, and both Round and Green Lakes at Green Lakes State Park, page 58, are examples of this. If you want to view this process on a smaller scale, look at the potholes along the Gorge Trail at Buttermilk Falls State Park, page 157, or potholes along the Gorge Trail at Watkins Glen State Park, page 194.

The enormity of the ice and its power to alter the landscape are hard to grasp, but the trails featured in this book are all evidence of its passage. Experienced individually the trails are interesting and illustrative, but I encourage you to take this knowledge and perspective (and, of course, this guidebook) while exploring all of the trails and find that common thread and awe for yourself. In the end, the book is about the landscape left behind by these great sheets of ice.

Book Divisions and Regions

WHILE I WAS RESEARCHING and selecting trails for the book, one thing became very obvious: Hiking trails are not evenly distributed across the region. They are often clustered near one another and possess similar characteristics. Based on the natural history of the area, this would be expected (that is, where the ice stalled, it altered the terrain a certain way, and where it mostly moved, it bulldozed the landscape differently). For example, in the south there are more hanging valleys and deeply cut gorges related to the Valley Heads Moraine and the formation of the great glacial lakes behind it. To the north, different processes led to the formation of the plunge pool lakes, hummocky topography, and drumlins. But what truly divides the region is literally the heart of the matter: the Finger Lakes themselves. Other than by boat, there is no way across the long sinuous Finger Lakes. To reach the opposing shore of each lake, you must drive the entire length of the lake. It's no surprise that most major highways circumnavigate the lakes, and the easiest and fastest routes through the region avoid this center. Don't get me wrong; the easiest route is by no means the most scenic. The north-south roads that follow each lake are some of the most picturesque in the region and are a major attraction, most notably for the numerous wineries and related wine trails that follow these roads. So a natural division of the area placed the Finger Lakes at the center, and the region is divided along the cardinal points roughly around them.

North

This area lies to the north of I-90 and includes all of the trails that border Lake Ontario. Essentially a broad drumlin field that runs from Syracuse to Rochester, the landscape has a slightly more muted feel than the deeply scoured gorges and pothole lakes that characterize other regions. But its excellent wildlife viewing and the oceanlike panoramas along Lake Ontario make up for its lack of waterfalls and gorges. Migration season and the height of summer are prime times to visit this part of the state.

East

I-81 is the major route through this region, and the interstate follows what is essentially a filled-in finger lake. Similar to the Finger Lakes to the west, an old river valley was deeply scoured and the hills were oversteepened. But as the ice sheet receded, the terminal moraine that helped form the lakes to the west did not block the flow of water to form a finger lake in this U-shaped valley. Woodlands, pothole lakes, and lovely hanging waterfalls are highlighted here. In the eastern region, the Finger Lakes Trail and North Country Trail head off in their separate ways: The former heads southeast toward the Catskills, while the latter heads northeast toward the Adirondacks.

South

Most of the trails in the southern area showcase the most striking examples of the lasting effects the past ice age had. Hanging valleys, deeply cut gorges, and iconic waterfalls are heavily featured here, but there are also deep woodlands for those who eschew crowds or are looking for more-challenging hikes. The area sprawls from Watkins Glen at the southern tip of Seneca Lake to Ithaca at the southern tip of Cayuga Lake and includes many of the state parks and most dramatic waterscapes in the book.

West

The smaller Finger Lakes are found along the western section of the region. The area is also farthest from major and even minor cities, so seclusion is almost guaranteed when compared with the crowds at the iconic state parks found elsewhere. Centered on Naples and the area around Canandaigua Lake, trails in this part of the state often incorporate a section of the Bristol Hills Trails, a north-south spur along the Finger Lakes Trail.

How to Use This Guidebook

THE FOLLOWING INFORMATION walks you through this guidebook's organization to make it easy and convenient for planning great hikes.

Overview Map, Map Key, & Map Legend

The overview map on the inside front cover depicts the location of
the primary trailhead for all 37 of the hikes described in this book.
The numbers shown on the overview map pair with the map key on
page i. Each hike's number remains with that hike throughout the
book. Thus, if you spot an appealing hiking area on the overview
map, you can flip through the book and find those hikes easily by
their sequential numbers at the top of each profile page.

Trail Maps

In addition to the overview map on the inside cover, a detailed
map of each hike's route appears with its profile. On each of these
maps, symbols indicate the trailhead, the complete route, significant
features, facilities, and topographic landmarks such as creeks,
overlooks, and peaks. A legend identifying the map symbols used
throughout the book appears on the inside back cover.

To produce the highly accurate maps in this book, the author
used a handheld GPS unit to gather data while hiking each route, and
then sent that data to the publisher's expert cartographers. However,
your GPS is not really a substitute for sound, sensible navigation that
takes into account the conditions that you observe while hiking.

Further, despite the high quality of the maps in this guidebook,
the publisher and author strongly recommend that you always carry
an additional map, such as the ones noted in each entry opener's list-
ing for "Maps."

Elevation Profile (Diagram)

For trails with any significant elevation changes, the hike description
will include this profile graph. Entries for fairly flat routes, such as a
lake loop, will *not* display an elevation profile.

Also, each entry's opener will list the elevation at the hike trailhead, and it will list the elevation peak.

For hike descriptions where the elevation profile is included,
this diagram represents the rises and falls of the trail as viewed from

the side, over the complete distance (in miles) of that trail. On the diagram's vertical axis, or height scale, the number of feet indicated between each tick mark lets you visualize the climb. To avoid making flat hikes look steep and steep hikes appear flat, varying height scales provide an accurate image of each hike's climbing challenge. For example, one hike's scale might rise to 500 feet, while another goes to 2,200 feet.

The Hike Profile

Each profile opens with the hike's star ratings, GPS trailhead coordinates, and other key at-a-glance information—from the trail's distance and configuration to contacts for local information. Each profile also includes a map (see "Trail Maps," page 7). The main text for each profile includes four sections: "Overview," "Route Details," "Nearby Attractions," and "Directions" (for driving to the trailhead area). Explanations of each of these elements follow.

Star Ratings

Five-Star Trails is the title of a Menasha Ridge Press guidebook series geared to specific cities/regions across the United States, such as this one for the Finger Lakes and Central New York. Following is the explanation for the rating system of one to five stars in five different categories for each hike.

FOR SCENERY:

★★★★★ Unique, picturesque panoramas

★★★★ Diverse vistas

★★★ Pleasant views

★★ Unchanging landscape

★ Not selected for scenery

FOR TRAIL CONDITION:

★★★★★ Consistently well maintained

★★★★ Stable, with no surprises

★★★ Average terrain to negotiate

★★ Inconsistent, with good and poor areas

★ Rocky, overgrown, or often muddy

FOR CHILDREN:

★★★★★ Babes in strollers are welcome

★★★★ Fun for anyone past the toddler stage

★★★ Good for young hikers with proven stamina

★★ Not enjoyable for children

★ Not advisable for children

FOR DIFFICULTY:

★★★★★ Grueling

★★★★ Strenuous

★★★ Moderate (won't beat you up—but you'll know you've been hiking)

★★ Easy with patches of moderate

★ Good for a relaxing stroll

FOR SOLITUDE:

★★★★★ Positively tranquil

★★★★ Spurts of isolation

★★★ Moderately secluded

★★ Crowded on weekends and holidays

★ Steady stream of individuals and/or groups

Key At-a-Glance Information

GPS TRAILHEAD COORDINATES

As noted in "Trail Maps" (see page 7), the author used a handheld GPS unit to obtain geographic data and sent the information to the publisher's cartographers. In the opener for each hike profile, the coordinates—the intersection of the latitude (north) and longitude (west)—will orient you from the trailhead. In some cases, you can drive within viewing distance of a trailhead. Other hiking routes require a short walk to the trailhead from a parking area.

You will also note that this guidebook uses the degree–decimal minute format for presenting the latitude and longitude GPS coordinates. The latitude and longitude grid system is likely quite familiar to you, but here is a refresher, pertinent to visualizing the GPS coordinates:

Imaginary lines of latitude—called parallels and approximately 69 miles apart from each other—run horizontally around the globe. The equator is established to be 0°, and each parallel is indicated by degrees from the equator: up to 90°N at the North Pole, and down to 90°S at the South Pole.

Imaginary lines of longitude—called meridians—run perpendicular to latitude lines. Longitude lines are likewise indicated by degrees. Starting from 0° at the Prime Meridian in Greenwich, England, they continue to the east and west until they meet 180° later at the International Date Line in the Pacific Ocean. At the equator, longitude lines also are approximately 69 miles apart, but that distance narrows as the meridians converge toward the North and South Poles.

To convert GPS coordinates given in degrees, minutes, and seconds to the format used here in degrees–decimal minutes, the seconds are divided by 60. For more on GPS technology, visit **usgs.gov.**

DISTANCE & CONFIGURATION

Distance notes the length of the hike round-trip, from start to finish. If the hike description includes options to shorten or extend the hike, those round-trip distances will also be factored here. Configuration defines the trail as a loop, an out-and-back (taking you in and out via the same route), a figure eight, or a balloon.

HIKING TIME

While researching the book, I had a typical hiking pace of 4–5 miles an hour. These paces were considerably faster than when I hiked the trails featured in my Adirondack book and reflect the relatively flat character of the trails in this region. This pace was on the fast side and required a concerted effort to maintain. I feel that the typical 3 miles an hour is a more suitable hiking pace to allow you to enjoy the hike, but experienced and conditioned hikers will use slightly faster paces. I've tried to base the time recommendations on a reasonable hiking pace while also including time to enjoy scenic views or, on longer hikes, to stop and rest. When deciding whether or not to follow a particular trail in this guidebook, consider the weather along with your own pace, general physical condition, and energy level that day.

HIGHLIGHTS

Waterfalls, historic sites, or other features that draw hikers to the trail are emphasized here.

ELEVATION

In each trail's opener, you will see the elevation at the trailhead and another figure for the peak height on the route. For routes that entail significant inclines and declines, the full hike profile also includes a complete elevation profile (see page 7).

ACCESS

Fees or permits required to hike the trail are detailed here—and noted if there are none. Trail-access hours are also shown.

MAPS

Resources for maps, in addition to those in this guidebook, are listed here. (As previously noted, the publisher and author recommend that you carry more than one map—and that you consult those maps before heading out on the trail to resolve any confusion or discrepancy.) Common abbreviations listed here include DEC for Department of Environmental Conservation, FLT for Finger Lakes Trail, and USGS for United States Geological Survey.

FACILITIES

This section alerts you to restrooms, phones, water, picnic tables, and other basics at or near the trailhead.

WHEELCHAIR ACCESS

At a glance, you'll see if there are paved sections or other areas for safely using a wheelchair.

COMMENTS

Here you will find assorted nuggets of information, such as whether or not dogs are allowed on the trails.

CONTACTS

Listed here are phone numbers and website addresses for checking trail conditions and gleaning other day-to-day information.

Overview, Route Details, Nearby Attractions, & Directions

These four elements provide the main text about the hike. "Overview" gives you a quick summary of what to expect on that trail; the "Route Details" guide you on the hike, start to finish; and "Nearby Attractions" will suggest appealing area sites, such as restaurants, museums, and other trails. "Directions" should get you to the trailhead from a well-known road or highway.

Weather

SPRING IS PROBABLY THE MOST PROBLEMATIC of the seasons for planning a trip. Many trails are still closed due to the need to clean up after winter and/or the potential for flooding. Likewise spring brings mud along all but the most developed of trails. Snow is known to fall as late as May, which means being prepared for cold weather is a must. During the spring melt the waterfalls are at their fullest and most dramatic, so you'll want to make a trip to one of the gorges and/or waterfalls as soon as safe and possible. Unfortunately this is also around the time black flies are likely, so plan accordingly. Because wildlife is on the move at this time of year, birding at the management areas and preserves should also be a focus. Late spring and early summer are the best times to catch trillium in bloom. If you choose one of the forest trails, you might be welcomed by carpets of these unique white flowers that are brief in their flowering and come out only before the trees leaf out, typically in late May.

In my opinion, summer is second only to fall for hiking seasons, and you really can't go wrong enjoying any of the trails throughout the summer. The forest trails offer a welcome reprieve from the region's high humidity; often a few degrees cooler, these shaded trails provide some relief from summer heat. Trails will often be dry, but so too will the seasonal streams. With swimming available at many of the state park trails listed, cooling off after a hike is easy should you choose to visit one of these. Unfortunately the height of summer is also when most of the waterfall trails are at their lowest. The winds off of Lake Ontario make the trails along its shore an ideal choice during summer.

In fall the forests are ablaze with color and those few trails that offer panoramic views will be well worth the effort. Crisp air and the crunching of leaves underfoot make autumn one of my favorite times to go hiking, but the falling of the leaves also heralds the start of hunting season. Plan your woodland excursions early in autumn so that you can take in the colors at their peak and limit your exposure to bow hunters. As the season comes to an end, many of the gorge trails will close and most woodland trails will begin to take on a new character. You have only a few short weeks to enjoy the altering appearance of these trails before snowshoes become essential gear.

During the winter, the state park gorge trails are closed, but hiking—or rather snowshoeing or cross-country skiing—along the forest trails offers a whole new perspective and beauty. Snow for these activities is typically best in late January or February once the base has compacted enough to support your weight. But as any upstate resident knows, lake-effect snows can blanket the area with feet of snow on any given day or week throughout the winter. Late dusks and early dawns will mean tightening your schedule and deducting 1 mile per hour from your typical hiking pace.

The following chart lists average temperatures and precipitation by month for the Finger Lakes and Central New York region. For each month, "Hi Temp" is the average daytime high; "Lo Temp" is the average nighttime low; and "Rain" is the average precipitation.

MONTH	HI TEMP	LO TEMP	RAIN
January	32°F	16°F	2.12"
February	34°F	18°F	1.98"
March	43°F	24°F	2.69"
April	56°F	35°F	3.22"
May	68°F	45°F	3.14"

MONTH	HI TEMP	LO TEMP	RAIN
June	77°F	55°F	3.70"
July	81°F	60°F	3.81"
August	79°F	58°F	3.51"
September	72°F	51°F	3.61"
October	60°F	40°F	3.32"
November	48°F	33°F	3.17"
December	37°F	23°F	2.56"

Water

THOUGH MANY OF THE TRAILS are in rural areas, few, if any, could truly be considered wilderness areas. So besides the risks of giardia (described below) found in most wilderness settings, a secondary and perhaps more pressing concern would be runoff from neighboring farms and/or civilized areas. Many of the trails are surrounded by civilization, and the chemicals and runoff from livestock are just as hazardous and unappetizing as drinking out of a puddle along a city street. Runoff can come from miles away, and the simplest way to prepare for this is not to plan on drinking water from sources found along the trail. Most trails featured in this book are not long enough or remote enough that finding water would be a realistic need. Instead my advice is to hydrate before setting out, carry enough for your thirst along the trail (approximately 6 ounces per mile), and have something in your vehicle for when you get off the trail. But remember that on a hot summer day, while a chilled bottle of water waiting at the car is a pleasant reward, it is of little use when you need it most along the trail. For most people, the pleasures of hiking make carrying water a relatively minor price to pay for remaining safe and healthy. So pack more water than you anticipate needing even for short hikes.

If you are tempted to drink "found" water, do so with extreme caution. Maps provided by the Finger Lakes Trail Conference often note reliable sources of water for long-distance hikers, and you should look for these sources before resorting to other "found" sources. Many ponds and lakes encountered by hikers are fairly stagnant and the water tastes terrible. Drinking such water presents inherent risks for thirsty trekkers besides the aforementioned issues with runoff. Giardia parasites contaminate many water sources and cause the dreaded intestinal giardiasis that can last for weeks after ingestion. For information, visit the Centers for Disease Control website at **cdc.gov /parasites/giardia.**

In any case, effective treatment is essential before using any water source found along the trail. Boiling water for 2–3 minutes is always a safe measure for camping, but day hikers can consider iodine tablets, approved chemical mixes, filtration units rated for giardia, and UV filtration. Some of these methods (for example, filtration with an added carbon filter) remove bad tastes typical in stagnant water, while others add their own taste. As a precaution, carry a means of water purification to help in a pinch and if you realize you have underestimated your consumption needs.

Clothing

WEATHER, UNEXPECTED TRAIL CONDITIONS, fatigue, extended hiking duration, and wrong turns can individually or collectively turn a great outing into a very uncomfortable one at best—and a life-threatening one at worst. Thus, proper attire plays a key role in helping you stay comfortable and, sometimes, alive. Here are some helpful guidelines:

★ Choose silk, wool, or synthetics for maximum comfort in all of your hiking attire—from hats to socks and in between. Cotton is fine if the weather remains dry and stable, but you won't be happy if that material gets wet.

★ Always wear a hat, or at least tuck one into your day pack or hitch it to your belt. Hats offer all-weather sun and wind protection as well as warmth if it turns cold.

★ Be ready to layer up or down as the day progresses and the mercury rises or falls. Today's outdoor wear makes layering easy, with such designs as jackets that convert to vests and zip-off or button-up legs.

★ Wear hiking boots or sturdy hiking sandals with toe protection. Flip-flopping along a paved urban greenway is one thing, but never hike a trail in open sandals or casual sneakers. Your bones and arches need support, and your skin needs protection.

★ Pair that footwear with good socks! If you prefer not to sheathe your feet when wearing hiking sandals, tuck the socks into your day pack; you may need them if the weather plummets or if you hit rocky turf and pebbles begin to irritate your feet. And, in an emergency, if you have lost your gloves, you can adapt the socks into mittens.

★ Don't leave raingear behind, even if the day dawns clear and sunny. Tuck into your day pack, or tie around your waist, a jacket that is breathable and either water-resistant or waterproof. Investigate different choices at your local outdoors retailer. If you are a frequent hiker, ideally you'll have more than one raingear weight, material, and style in your closet to protect you in all seasons in your regional climate and hiking microclimates.

Essential Gear

TODAY YOU CAN BUY OUTDOOR VESTS that have up to 20 pockets shaped and sized to carry everything from toothpicks to binoculars. Or, if you don't aspire to feel like a burro, you can neatly stow all of these items in your day pack or backpack. The following list showcases never-hike-without-them items, in alphabetical order, as all are important:

★ *Extra food* (trail mix, granola bars, or other high-energy foods)

★ *Extra clothes* (raingear, warm hat, gloves, and change of socks and shirt)

★ *Flashlight or headlamp* with extra bulb and batteries

★ *Insect repellent* (For some areas and seasons, this is extremely vital.)

★ *Maps and a high-quality compass* (Even if you know the terrain from previous hikes, don't leave home without these tools. And, as previously noted, bring maps in addition to those in this guidebook, and consult them prior to the hike. If you are versed in GPS usage, bring that device too, but don't rely on it as your sole navigational tool. Its battery life can dwindle or die, and be sure to compare its guidance with that of your maps.)

★ *Pocketknife and/or multitool*

★ *Sunscreen* (Note the expiration date on the tube or bottle; it's usually embossed on the top.)

★ *Water* (As emphasized more than once in this book, bring more than you think you will drink. Depending on your destination, you may want to bring a container and iodine or a filter for purifying water in case you run out.)

★ *Whistle* (This little gadget will be your best friend in an emergency.)

★ *Windproof matches* and/or a lighter, as well as a fire starter

First-Aid Kit

In addition to the items above, those below may appear overwhelming for a day hike. But any paramedic will tell you that the products listed here—in alphabetical order, because all are important—are just the basics. The reality of hiking is that you can be out for a week of backpacking and acquire only a mosquito bite. Or you can hike for an hour, slip, and suffer a bleeding abrasion or broken bone. Fortunately, these listed items will collapse into a very small space. You also may purchase convenient, prepackaged kits at your pharmacy or on the Internet.

★ Ace bandages or Spenco joint wraps

★ Antibiotic ointment (Neosporin or the generic equivalent)

★ Athletic tape

★ Band-Aids

★ Benadryl or the generic equivalent diphenhydramine (in case of allergic reactions)

★ Blister kit (such as Moleskin/Spenco Second Skin)

★ Butterfly-closure bandages

★ Epinephrine in a prefilled syringe (typically by prescription only, and for people known to have severe allergic reactions to hiking occurrences such as bee stings)

★ Gauze (one roll and a half dozen 4-by-4-inch pads)

★ Hydrogen peroxide or iodine

★ Ibuprofen or acetaminophen

Note: Consider your intended terrain and the number of hikers in your party before you exclude any article cited above. A botanical garden stroll may not inspire you to carry a complete kit, but anything beyond that warrants precaution. When hiking alone, you should always be prepared for a medical need. And if you are a twosome or with a group, one or more people in your party should be equipped with first-aid material.

General Safety

The following tips may have the familiar ring of your mother's voice as you take note of them.

★ *Always let someone know where you will be hiking* and how long you expect to be gone. It's a good idea to give that person a copy of your route, particularly if you are headed into any isolated area. Let them know when you return.

★ *Always sign in and out of any trail registers provided.* Don't hesitate to comment on the trail condition if space is provided; that's your opportunity to alert others to any problems you encounter.

★ *Do not count on a cell phone for your safety.* Reception may be spotty or nonexistent on the trail, even on an urban walk—especially if it is embraced by towering trees.

★ *Always carry food and water,* even for a short hike. And bring more water than you think you will need. (That cannot be said often enough!)

★ *Ask questions.* State forest and park employees are there to help. It's a lot easier to solicit advice before a problem occurs, and it will help you avoid a mishap away from civilization when it's too late to amend an error.

★ *Stay on designated trails.* Even on the most clearly marked trails, there is usually a point where you have to stop and consider which direction to head. If you become disoriented, don't panic. As soon as you think you may be off track, stop, assess your current direction, and then retrace your steps to the point where you went astray. Using a map, a compass, and this book, and keeping in mind what you have passed thus far, reorient yourself and trust your judgment on which way to continue. If you become absolutely unsure of how to continue, return to your vehicle the way you came in. Should you become completely lost and have no idea how to find the trailhead, remaining in place along the trail and waiting for help is most often the best option for adults and always the best option for children.

★ *Always carry a whistle,* another precaution that cannot be over-emphasized. It may be a lifesaver if you do become lost or sustain an injury.

★ *Be especially careful when crossing streams.* Whether you are ford-ing the stream or crossing on a log, make every step count. If you have any doubt about maintaining your balance on a log, ford the stream instead: use a trekking pole or stout stick for balance *and face upstream as you cross.* If a stream seems too deep to ford, turn back. Whatever is on the other side is not worth risking your life.

★ *Be careful at overlooks.* While these areas may provide spectacular views, they are potentially hazardous. Stay back from the edge of outcrops, and make absolutely sure of your footing; a misstep can mean a nasty and possibly fatal fall.

★ *Standing dead trees and storm-damaged living trees pose a signifi-cant hazard to hikers.* These trees may have loose or broken limbs that could fall at any time. While walking beneath trees, and when choosing a spot to rest or enjoy your snack, look up!

★ *Know the symptoms of subnormal body temperature known as hypo-thermia.* Shivering and forgetfulness are the two most common indi-cators of this stealthy killer. Hypothermia can occur at any elevation, even in the summer, especially when the hiker is wearing lightweight cotton clothing. If symptoms present themselves, get to shelter, hot liquids, and dry clothes ASAP.

★ *Know the symptoms of heat exhaustion (hyperthermia).* Lightheaded-ness and loss of energy are the first two indicators. If you feel these symptoms, find some shade, drink your water, remove as many lay-ers of clothing as practical, and stay put until you cool down. March-ing through heat exhaustion leads to heatstroke—which can be fatal. If you should be sweating and you're not, that's the signature warning sign. Your hike is over at that point—heatstroke is a life-threatening condition that can cause seizures, convulsions, and eventually death. If you or a companion reaches that point, do whatever can be done to cool the victim down and seek medical attention immediately.

★ *Most important of all, take along your brain.* A cool, calculating mind is the single most important asset on the trail. It allows you to think before you act.

★ *In summary:* Plan ahead. Watch your step. Avoid accidents before they happen. Enjoy a rewarding and relaxing hike.

Watchwords for Flora and Fauna

Hikers should remain aware of the following concerns regarding plant- and wildlife, described in alphabetical order.

BLACK BEARS: Black bears are found throughout New York State, but are most frequently encountered in the Adirondacks and occasionally in the Catskills. Though attacks by black bears are virtually unheard of, a bear tearing up your gear or rummaging about outside your tent will give anyone a start. If you encounter a bear at your campsite or while hiking, remain calm and never run away. Make loud noises to scare off the bear and back away slowly. Most of the trails in state parks are too built up, small, and/or isolated to support bears, but the trails within state forests are another matter. In primitive and remote areas, assume that bears are present, and in more developed sites ask the park staff about the current bear situation. Most encounters are food related, as bears have an exceptional sense of smell and will eat everything. A clean site combined with care and caution will keep these foragers away from your campsite. Store all food, cooking equipment, and garbage in tightly sealed containers and place well away from your tent. In remote areas or those with recent bear activity, store all items in storage lockers or bear canisters, or suspend in a sack 12 feet above the ground, 6 feet below branches, and 12 feet from neighboring trees. Make sure that your site is clean and never leave food unattended. Clean your utensils and cooking equipment at least 100 feet from your site and never dump uneaten food on the ground. Do not bring food into your tent and do not sleep in clothes worn while preparing food. Generally, proper food preparation and garbage disposal will help maintain a pristine wilderness, the safety of bears and other wildlife, and an enjoyable camping experience for everyone.

BLACK FLIES: Though certainly a pest and maddening annoyance, the worst a black fly will cause is an itchy welt. They are most active from mid-May into June, during the day, and especially before thunderstorms, as well as during the morning and evening hours. Insect repellent has some effect, though the only way to avoid their swarming midst is to keep moving.

MOSQUITOES: You will encounter mosquitoes on most of the hikes described in this book. Insect repellent and/or repellent-impregnated clothing are the only simple methods to ward off these pests. Mosquitoes in New York are known to carry the West Nile virus, so all due caution should be taken to avoid mosquito bites.

POISON IVY, OAK, & SUMAC: Recognizing and avoiding poison ivy, oak, and sumac are the most effective ways to prevent the painful, itchy rashes associated with these plants. Poison ivy occurs as a vine or ground cover, three leaflets to a leaf; poison oak occurs as either a vine or shrub, also with three leaflets; and poison sumac flourishes in swampland, each leaf having 7–13 leaflets. Urushiol, the oil in the sap of these plants, is responsible for the rash. Within 14 hours of exposure, raised lines and/or blisters will appear on the affected area, accompanied by a terrible itch. Refrain from scratching, because bacteria under your fingernails can cause an infection. Wash and dry the affected area thoroughly, applying a calamine lotion to help dry out the rash. If itching or blistering is severe, seek medical attention. If you do come into contact with one of these plants, remember that oil-contaminated clothes, hiking gear, and pets can easily cause an irritating rash on you or someone else, so wash not only any exposed parts of your body but also any exposed clothes, gear, and pets.

SNAKES: New York has a variety of snakes—including garter, milk, and water snakes—most of which are benign. Timber rattlesnakes, northern copperhead, and eastern massasauga rattlesnakes are the exceptions, though they dwell primarily in very isolated areas. According to the Department of Environmental Conservation the massasauga is found in two isolated marshy areas: one near Syracuse and the other near Rochester. The copperhead is mostly found along the Hudson Valley but is largely absent from the Catskills. The timber rattlesnake is the most widely dispersed of the three and is found in rugged deciduous forests along the southern edge of the state and up into the eastern Adirondacks. Encounters with any of these species are very rare and virtually impossible along the trails of Central New York and the Finger Lakes.

TICKS: Ticks are often found on brush and tall grass waiting to hitch a ride on a warm-blooded passerby. Adult ticks are most active in the New York area between April and May and again between October and November. Among the local varieties of ticks, the black-legged tick, commonly called the deer tick, is the primary carrier of Lyme disease. You can use several strategies to reduce your chances of ticks getting under your skin. Some people choose to wear light-colored clothing, so ticks can be spotted before they make it to the skin. Most important, be sure to visually check hair, back of neck, armpits, and socks at the end of the hike. During your post-hike shower, take a moment to do a more complete body check. For ticks that are already embedded, removal with tweezers is best. Use disinfectant solution on the wound.

TOURISTS: While unavoidable at some of the more spectacular trails, tourists can be avoided by choosing to hike during off-hours and off-seasons. However, do try to remember that if you seem to be surrounded by them and you are not in your house, well, then, you are in fact one of them.

Hunting

Separate rules, regulations, and licenses govern the various hunting types and related seasons. Among the trails featured in the book, some prohibit hunting entirely, while others allow limited hunting or only in special areas along or near the trails. As a general guideline hunting is usually very limited in state parks and preserves while more common in state forests and wildlife management areas. I've noted places where hunting is more common, but always check during the seasons listed below. The opening weekends tend to be when the woods suddenly fill with orange and camouflage, so for those few days it's probably best to choose one of the areas where hunting is prohibited. Below is a general outline of the hunting seasons in Central New York and the Finger Lakes.

★ Archery Season (Deer): Early October to opening of regular season. One week following regular season.

★ Turkey: Early October to regular deer season.

★ Regular Season (Deer): Mid-November–mid-December.

Specific start dates are available on the Department of Environmental Conservation website: **dec.ny.gov/outdoor/65231.html.**

Regulations

The rules and regulations regarding the use and activities along the trails vary widely. Though I've tried to note regulations that typically coincide with hiking, you should always check with the regulating agency before visiting if you plan on doing anything beyond hiking the trails or when in doubt.

The trails featured in the book traverse a wide variety of properties, including federal, state, county, and private lands. To simplify things, it is easiest to group the trails as either within parks and preserves or within forests and wildlife management areas. Parks and preserves would include most of the trails found within state and county parks, land trust preserves, and private land. These have the widest variety of managing agencies, each with their own rules and regulations. Furthermore, each regulating agency may have different rules for different parks, so you should check with the local contacts provided regarding activities allowed. For the most part, these areas are the most restrictive about the what, when, and where of activities allowed. Generally speaking, trails within these areas typically prohibit the building of fires, except perhaps in grills or fire rings; have specific access requirements (such as fees, limited hours, or designated parking areas); have designated swimming areas; and prohibit camping along the trails or in the park except in designated campgrounds (see *Best Tent Camping: New York State* for recommendations).

On the other hand, activities within state forests and wildlife management areas are the least restrictive and allow for a wider variety of outdoor activities, typically free, year-round, and 24/7. These areas offer the least in the way of amenities and the closest to a wilderness experience as possible. These properties are managed by the Department of Environmental Conservation, and their rules and regulations are good advice for most hikers, so I've outlined them below.

★ Camping is prohibited within 150 feet of any road, trail, spring, stream, pond, or other body of water except at areas designated by a "Camp Here" disk.

★ Groups of 10 or more persons OR stays of more than three days in one place require a permit from the New York State Forest Ranger responsible for the area.

★ Lean-tos are available in many areas on a first-come, first-serve basis. Lean-tos cannot be used exclusively and must be shared with other campers.

★ Use pit privies provided near popular camping areas and trailheads. If none are available, dispose of human waste by digging a hole 6–8 inches deep at least 150 feet from water or campsites. Cover with leaves and soil.

★ Do not use soap to wash yourself, clothing, or dishes within 150 feet of water.

★ Drinking and cooking water should be boiled for 5 minutes, treated with purifying tablets, or filtered through a filtration device to prevent instances of giardia infection.

★ Fires should be built in existing fire pits or fireplaces if provided. Use only dead and down wood for fires. Cutting standing trees is prohibited. Extinguish all fires with water and stir ashes until they are cold to the touch. Do not build fires in areas marked by a "No Fires" disk. Camp stoves are safer, more efficient, and cleaner.

★ Carry out what you carry in. Practice "Leave No Trace" camping and hiking.

★ Keep your pet under control. Restrain it on a leash when others approach. Collect and bury droppings away from water, trails, and campsites. Keep your pet away from drinking water sources.

★ Observe and enjoy wildlife and plants, but leave them undisturbed.

★ Removing plants, rocks, fossils, or artifacts from state land without a permit is illegal.

Trail Etiquette

Always treat the trail, wildlife, and fellow hikers with respect. Here are some reminders.

★ Plan ahead to be self-sufficient at all times. For example, carry necessary supplies for changes in weather or other conditions. A well-planned trip brings satisfaction to you and to others.

★ Hike on open trails only.

★ In seasons or construction areas where road or trail closures may be a possibility, use the website addresses or phone numbers shown in the "Contacts" line for each of this guidebook's hikes to check conditions prior to heading out for your hike. And do not attempt to circumvent such closures.

★ Avoid trespassing on private land, and obtain all permits and authorization as required. Also, leave gates as you found them or as directed by signage.

★ Be courteous to hikers, bikers, equestrians, and others you encounter on the trails.

★ Never spook wild animals or pets. An unannounced approach, a sudden movement, or a loud noise startles most critters, and a surprised animal can be dangerous to you, to others, and to itself. Give animals plenty of space.

★ Observe the yield signs around the region's trailheads and backcountry. Typically they advise hikers to yield to horses, and bikers yield to both horses and hikers. By common courtesy on hills, hikers and bikers yield to any uphill traffic. When encountering mounted riders or horse packers, hikers can courteously step off the trail, on the downhill side if possible. So the horse can see and hear you, calmly greet the riders before they reach you and do not dart behind trees. Also resist the urge to pet horses unless you are invited to do so.

★ Stay on the existing trail and do not blaze any new trails.

★ Be sure to pack out what you pack in, leaving only your footprints. No one likes to see the trash someone else has left behind.

Tips on Enjoying Hiking in the Finger Lakes and Central New York

★ Many state parks grant free access if you purchase access to another state park on the same day, so plan to visit multiple parks nearby to save on fees.

★ With the purchase of an Empire Passport, you gain unlimited access to all of the New York state parks for one year.

★ Many state parks allow access but do not charge fees in late fall and winter. However, the off-season is also when the most scenic portions of the parks are closed for your safety (for example, gorge trails).

★ Gorge trails open in the spring, after maintenance and repairs from winter and flooding damage are complete. Because the amount of damage varies year to year, check with these parks before visiting to see if a trail is open to avoid a wasted trip.

★ State parks are busiest during the summer, when schools are not in session, but they are typically open a few weeks before and after the summer vacation. Trips during these off-seasons or during the week are the best ways to avoid crowds.

★ Waterfall trails are at their most dramatic during the spring melt and after heavy rains, so plan trips to these marvels after these events.

★ Each Finger Lake has its own wine trail, with vineyard tasting rooms along the length of the lakes. Many are nearby the trails featured, so check a map to add this other taste of the Finger Lakes to your trip. Tastings are offered through the late spring, summer, and early fall.

★ Fall is a favorite and scenic time of year to go hiking, but in Central New York, it is also apple season. Many orchards have apple-picking and other outdoor activities, and roadside stands offer fresh apple pies and other local produce and delicacies to hungry travelers.

★ One way to turn an out-and-back hike into a more interesting adventure is to leave a bike on one end of the trail (don't forget to bring your bike lock key) and ride back to your car.

★ Forest trails offer cooling shade in summer, but after the leaves have fallen in autumn, these trails reveal more scenic views, so plan on revisiting these hikes in fall and winter as well.

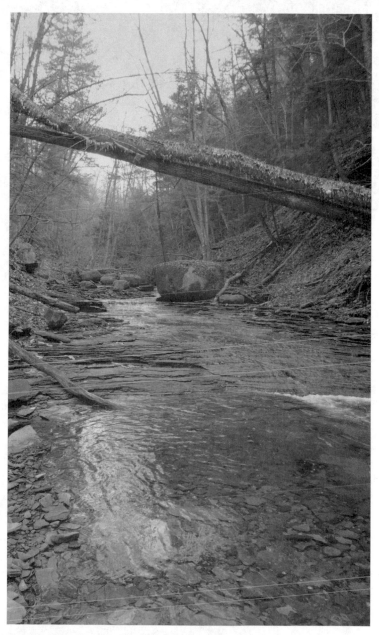

TRAIL 33 BRIGGS GULLY AT WESLEY HILL NATURE PRESERVE *see page 243*

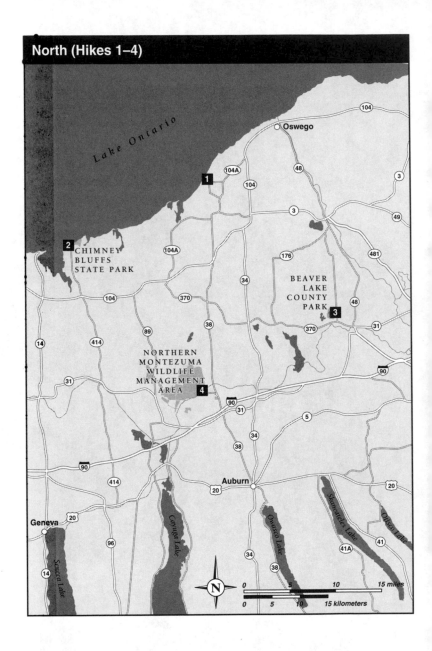

North (Hikes 1–4)

North

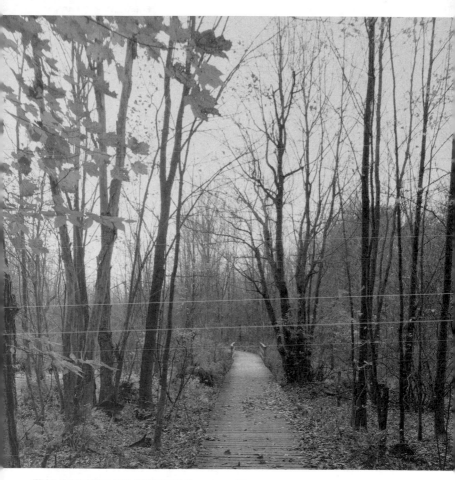

TRAIL 3 BEAVER LAKE BOARDWALK *see page 43*

Sterling Nature Center

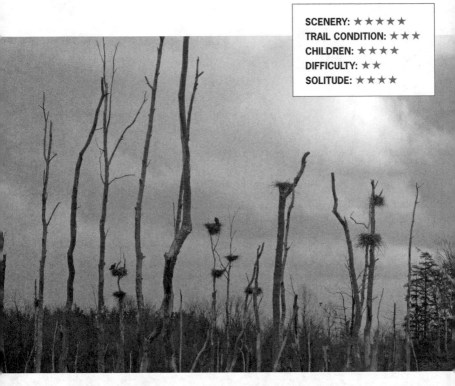

SCENERY: ★ ★ ★ ★
TRAIL CONDITION: ★ ★ ★
CHILDREN: ★ ★ ★ ★
DIFFICULTY: ★ ★
SOLITUDE: ★ ★ ★

GPS TRAILHEAD COORDINATES: N43° 22.722'   W76° 39.442'

DISTANCE & CONFIGURATION: 4.4-mile double figure eight; additional side trips available

HIKING TIME: 1.5–2 hours

HIGHLIGHTS: Panoramic views of Lake Ontario, wetlands, abundant birding and wildlife

ELEVATION: 310' at trailhead, with no significant change in elevation

ACCESS: Daily, sunrise–sunset; no fees or permits required

MAPS: Sterling Nature Center: **cayugacounty.us/livingworking/parksandtrails /sterling/mapsanddirections**; also available at park

FACILITIES: Interpretive center, store

WHEELCHAIR ACCESS: No

COMMENTS: Dogs must be on leash. The marsh here has an abundance of wildlife and birding opportunities, and I highly recommend that you bring a pair of binoculars.

CONTACTS: Sterling Nature Center, 315-947-6143, **cayugacounty.us/livingworking /parksandtrails/sterling**

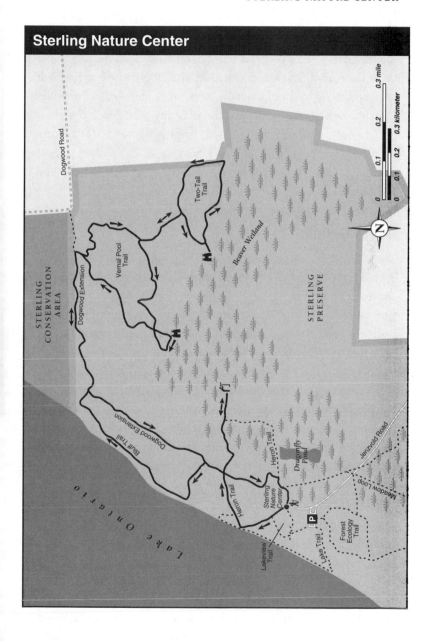

Overview

Mostly along level terrain, this trail system weaves among lake bluffs, quiet woodlands, and a sprawling wetland. The trail along the bluff has spectacular views of Lake Ontario, while the wetland provides some of the best birding opportunities of any of the trails described in this book. The wetland has a multitude of roosts for herons, ospreys, great horned owls, and even bald eagles. The rookery is most active May–July. To get the most out of your experience here, binoculars should be included in your packing list.

Route Details

The addition of new trails to the Sterling Nature Center, including a shoreline trail and a longer wetland loop, is currently being considered. However, at the time of this writing their implementation or completion date is unknown. Plan on including some extra time if you're fortunate to find that these trails have been completed before your visit. The route described below is a slightly odd configuration—two figure eights—but highlights much of what the park has to offer. Included in this configuration are the Lakeview Trail, a portion of the Heron Trail, the Bluff Trail, the Vernal Pool Trail, the Two-Tail Trail, and returning along the Dogwood Extension. From the large parking area, head toward the information kiosk, pick up a trail map, and continue up the road toward the nature center, where the trails begin and end.

Once behind the nature center, look to your left for the Lakeview Trail sign, a wood sign with orange lettering. The Lakeview Trail is a short loop trail (0.4 mile) near the center, and though the route described won't follow this trail, it shares its path very briefly to reach the Heron Trail. A green placard on a green post marks this intersection, and you should follow the Heron Trail, marked with blue dots, toward Lake Ontario. The trail follows an elevated path above the lake's rocky shoreline for a brief while before veering back eastward and away from the lake. There are many picturesque spots here, but even more await along the Bluff Trail farther along. In less than 0.25 mile, you reach an intersection with a gravel road. This is the Dogwood Extension, which serves as the main connecting trail for all the loops described. The route will return to this intersection shortly, but for now head straight across the road to follow the Heron Trail to the marsh observation deck.

The trail continues eastward beside a flat creek, the outlet of the marsh ahead. Shortly after crossing a tributary to this creek, the trail intersects the observation deck spur trail. The Heron Trail continues to the right, through an open field, and eventually back to the nature center. Bear left, essentially straight ahead and eastward, and in no time the spur ends at the observation deck. The broad marshland is the ideal setting for birding; herons, ospreys, great horned owls, and even bald eagles have been sighted here. Standing dead trees throughout the marsh are populated with numerous nests. Indeed, roosts seem to be everywhere; the counts vary from 60 to more than 90, and no doubt those who brought along binoculars will be amply rewarded. There is a lot to see here, but you'll encounter other vantage points of this wetland from the opposing shore later on.

Head back the way you came to the Dogwood Extension and turn right, northward, to continue the trail. You cross the creek over a large culvert and soon reach the intersection with the Bluff Trail on your left, at roughly 0.75 mile overall. The trail weaves westward, marked with brown paints, a little over 0.1 mile and then turns northward as sweeping views of Lake Ontario open before you. At times the wind coming off the lake can be quite strong, a welcome reprieve in summer but bitterly cold in fall and winter.

At 193 miles long and 53 miles wide, Lake Ontario has the smallest surface area (7,340 square miles) of the five Great Lakes. It is the fourth largest in volume and is the last of the lakes before the water flows into the Saint Lawrence River on its eventual path to the Atlantic Ocean. But the water has not always followed this course and may change yet again. Like the Finger Lakes, the Great Lakes were created during the Pleistocene ice age. Once the Ontarian River Valley, this valley was scoured by sheets of ice into a deep trough, and as the ice sheets retreated, their meltwater filled these deep basins to form immense lakes, even larger than those present today. During a period when the Saint Lawrence was still dammed by ice, an even larger lake, Lake Iroquois, existed. Its shore extended much farther than Ontario's does today, and its drainage flowed through what is now Syracuse and then eastward along the Mohawk River and into the Hudson. As the ice sheets retreated further, the Saint Lawrence outlet opened and the flow through its channel dominated. The removal of the great weight of ice has furthermore allowed the landscape to rebound and rise; the present uplift is about 1 foot per century. The land tilts ever southward, deepening the tributaries along the southern shore into estuaries, and it continues to do so. It is speculated that in millennia to come, the uplift will progress so far that Niagara Falls will cease to flow into Lake Ontario and the Great Lakes will eventually drain into the Mississippi.

The walk along the Bluff Trail is, in the Finger Lakes and Central New York, the closest thing to what it feels like hiking along an ocean. The scene is striking and picturesque all along the next 0.5 mile as the trail climbs gently northward along a narrow footpath. The trail turns sharply to the right, follows brown and occasional yellow paints east, and soon re-intersects with the Dogwood Extension.

Bear left at the intersection and head eastward along the broad road. Old maps show an intersecting trail that connects with the loops described elsewhere in this book, but this crossover trail is no longer maintained. The road passes through a wet area on both sides of the road—the northernmost area affected by the beaver wetland—and then climbs a short hill. A little over 0.3 mile along (1.75 miles overall), the road intersects the northern loops, the Vernal Pool and Two-Tail Trails, on your right. A large wooden sign with red lettering marks this intersection. Turn right and head south a very short distance; then bear left at the green placard indicating that the trail heads off in both directions. The trail is now marked with red paints and proceeds along the edge of the park boundary.

Less than 0.25 mile along this section, you intersect the Two-Tail Trail, marked with white paints, on your left. Proceed south over a short bridge and then reach what appears to be a sharp right turn in the trail. This is the beginning of the loop section along the Two-Tail Trail. However, without turning around or looking on the opposing side of the tree that marks the turn, you might mistake this for only a sharp turn in the trail and not the beginning of the loop. Had you mistook this simply as a turn, then later on when you reach the marsh, it may be confusing why you have not reached this intersection. Continue westward, to your right, though shortly ahead the trail bears left, southward, down a small hill, and you come into view of the beaver marsh. Had you missed the trail intersection previously, this may be a point that creates some confusion. The main trail turns to the left at this point, while to the right is a heavily trodden path to a marsh lookout—not a continuation of the trail. The lookout spur is unmarked and simply leads to points along the edge of the wetland where there are additional views of the marsh and its ample bird habitat. To follow the main trail, bear left and head eastward along the northern edge of the marsh, marked in white. In about 0.25 mile, the trail turns to the left and heads slightly uphill. You pass through a section of dense scrub and abandoned orchards and slowly weave your way back to the beginning of the loop, where, from this vantage point, the beginning of the loop is suddenly obvious.

Bear right and head back over the small bridge to reconnect with the Vernal Pool Trail, marked with red paints. Turn left at the intersection and head westward about 0.25 mile until you reach another trail intersection. To your left is a tiny loop, marked with red diamonds, which brings you to a vantage point of the marsh nearly directly across from the observation deck along the Heron loop. This extremely short loop will be your last chance to observe the marsh with its plethora of wildlife and photo ops. Back along the main loop, the trail begins to head northward and you encounter some larger vernal pools. Vernal pools are small woodland depressions that fill seasonally and provide an important source of water and breeding habitat for woodland amphibians. The pools by their nature are temporary, so whether you come upon the ones I observed will all depend on the season; spring is often the best time to observe them.

At 3.4 miles, you conclude the Vernal Pool circuit and shortly after reconnect with the Dogwood Extension. From here it is a little over a mile back to the nature center. As previously mentioned, the Dogwood Extension is an access road and pretty uneventful, so you might consider retracing your path if you desire some more scenery. In total, the trail described is almost 4.5 miles in length, but you should add ample time for photos and wildlife observation during your trip.

Nearby Attractions

Many people associate the town of Sterling with the summertime Sterling Renaissance Festival (**sterlingfestival.com**). Each weekend, from early July to mid-August, costumed entertainers, actors, comedians, and musicians reenact scenes reminiscent of the European Middle Ages. Also during the summer, a variety of weekend-long music festivals offers entertainment at the Sterling Stage (**sterling stage.com**). If you plan to extend your trip to enjoy these other activities, camping is available in the area at Fair Haven campgrounds described in *Best Tent Camping: New York State.*

Directions

From points east: From the intersections of NY 481 North and NY 3 West in Fulton, head west on NY 3/CR 3. Follow it 11.7 miles, and turn left on NY 104A. After 1 mile, turn right onto Center Road/CR 98. At 0.5 mile, stay left to continue on Center Road/CR 98. At 1.7 miles, turn right onto Macneil Road. Take the first left on CR 98/ Farden Road. At 1 mile, stay left on Jensvold Road and follow it to the parking area on the left, ahead 0.8 mile.

From points west: From I-90, take Exit 40. Turn left on NY 34 South, followed by a left onto NY 31 West/Erie Drive. At 4.3 miles, turn right onto NY 38 North/Canal Street. Follow NY 38 North for 20 miles into Sterling. Turn left onto Center Road/CR 98, and follow directions above.

Chimney Bluffs State Park

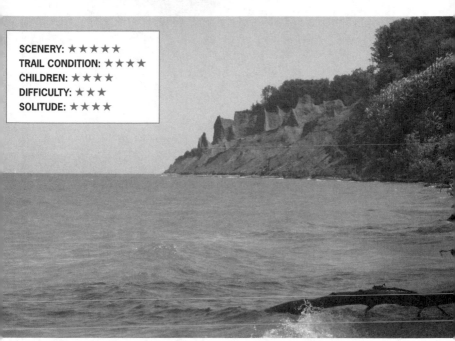

SCENERY: ★ ★ ★ ★ ★
TRAIL CONDITION: ★ ★ ★ ★
CHILDREN: ★ ★ ★ ★
DIFFICULTY: ★ ★ ★
SOLITUDE: ★ ★ ★ ★

GPS TRAILHEAD COORDINATES: (Main parking area) N43° 16.862'   W76° 55.347'
(East Bay Road parking area) N43° 17.399'   W76° 54.394'

DISTANCE & CONFIGURATION: 2.5-mile shoreline loop; 2.5-mile out-and-back

HIKING TIME: 1.5 hours

HIGHLIGHTS: Panoramic views, beachside stroll, geological features

ELEVATION: 250' at trailhead; 383' at highest point along bluff

ACCESS: Daily, sunrise–sunset; no fees or permits required

MAPS: NY State Park map: **nysparks.com/parks/43/maps.aspx**; USGS *Sodus Point*

FACILITIES: Restrooms, picnic benches

WHEELCHAIR ACCESS: Yes in the picnic area, but not along the trail

COMMENTS: Be careful around the trail edges along the bluffs. The area is actively erod-ing, and the ground near these edges may not be stable. Hikers have been injured in the past, so take caution along the rim. Dogs on a leash are allowed in the park but not recom-mended along the Bluff Trail due to unstable trail conditions along the rim.

CONTACTS: New York State Office of Parks, 315-947-5205, **nysparks.com/parks/43**

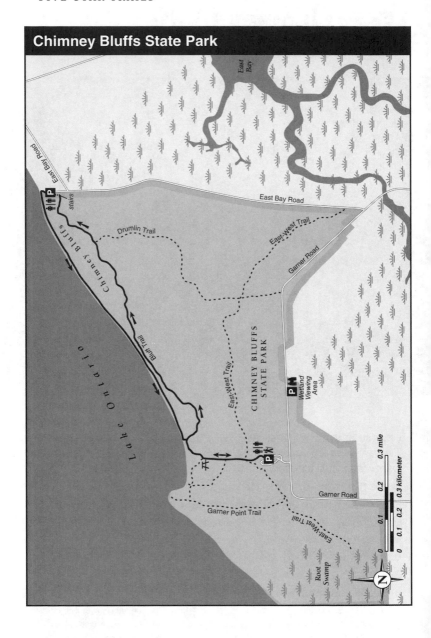

Chimney Bluffs State Park

Overview

Central New York is not known for its beaches or its coastal trails. How could it be? The region is hundreds of miles inland. Yet hiking the Chimney Bluffs trail makes you feel as if you are along one of the coasts. While the open views along Lake Ontario are certainly beautiful, the main attraction here are the bluffs. Formed from eroding drumlins, they create a must-see picturesque panorama.

Route Details

Unlike many state park trails featured in this book, there is no entrance fee associated with this trail. The state acquired this park in 1963, and there were plans to develop it similar to other parks across the state; but these plans were put aside and the park was left undeveloped until 1999. At that time, restrooms, trails, picnic areas with grills, and parking lots were built.

To find the trailhead from the parking area, head north along the paved walkway toward Lake Ontario. Continue past the picnic area, and you will see the Bluff Trail on your right as you approach the shoreline (approximately 0.25 mile from the parking area). You will begin heading east along a fairly broad trail, but as you delve deeper into the surrounding hardwoods, it dwindles to a narrow footpath.

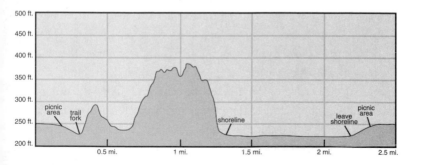

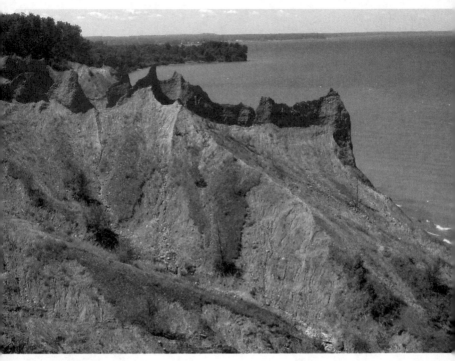

CHIMNEY BLUFFS

Blue diamonds mark the trail, but the way is pretty straightforward. The trail is mostly flat for the first 0.5 mile but soon begins to climb at approximately 0.6 mile in. The trail climbs 100 feet over the next 0.2 mile. Along the approach to the bluffs, occasional previews of the eroded drumlin ahead can be seen through the surrounding trees, but the truly breathtaking views don't begin until you reach the bluffs' rim a little shy of 1 mile into the hike. As the trail winds along the rim, be careful not to get too close to the edge, as steady erosion makes areas of this trail unstable. The chimneys/spires are spectacular and leave you wondering how they were formed and how long they will last.

Drumlins are a common geological feature of Central New York and were formed during the last glacial period some 12,000 years ago. As the glaciers made their long retreat north, they scoured the landscape and left streamlined hills of glacial deposits in their wake. These hills, known as drumlins, indicate the direction of the receding glaciers and are the common feature that defines the gentle hills and rolling valleys surrounding Syracuse and Rochester. The drumlins along Lake Ontario have been eroded by wind and water for millennia. On the shores of Chimney Bluffs State Park, heavy deposits of clay have provided a sticky mortar between cobbles and stones that have resisted the slow process of erosion and left an ever-changing landscape that is a spectacle to behold. The current rate of erosion is estimated to be 1–5 feet per year, and the whole area is in a constant state of change. There are many vantage points where you can observe this geological wonder, so take your time and enjoy the view, but beware of the unstable edges along the rim.

About 1 mile in, you intersect the Drumlin Trail on your right. You can use this trail, along with the East-West Trail, to provide a loop back to the parking area, but you will miss the pleasure of strolling along the shoreline at the bluffs' base. The Bluff Trail continues east and turns briefly northward, where a path off to the left offers a vantage point for looking back west at the bluffs. This side path weaves through some fairly unstable areas, so watch your step and stay away from the rim.

Past this point, the trail begins to descend toward the East Bay Road parking area and temporarily away from the bluffs. The descent becomes fairly steep, especially as the parking area comes into view. The trail switches back northward as it descends on the parking area. I hardly need to tell you to head toward the beach at this point because the lapping waters of the lakeshore will beckon you ahead. Indeed, many visitors proceed directly to this parking area because it provides a more direct route to the bluffs' base and Lake Ontario's shoreline.

Turn left and head west along the rocky shoreline. It doesn't take long before the chimneys and spires of the eroding drumlin tower above you. Lake Ontario spreads out across the northern horizon, and the unique setting of Chimney Bluffs really sets in. Few places in Central New York offer a similar experience, and that's why

I recommend this loop over the other prescribed trails. Stick to the shoreline and do not attempt to climb the unstable bluffs. The base of the bluffs is approximately 0.5 mile long, and soon after you will be walking within feet of the trail you began on, approximately 2 miles total. The shoreline is constantly changing, and you will have to keep an eye out for a convenient way to climb back onto the trail. Once back at the picnic area, return to the parking area, for a total trip length of 2.5 miles.

Nearby Attractions

Several other short trails are within the park's boundaries, but I chose to focus on the most dramatic loop available. For reference, the East-West Trail and Drumlin Trail can be combined with the Bluff Trail to create a loop of similar length, though these additional sections do not offer views or the additional attraction of walking along the shoreline.

Directions

Approximately 9 miles east of Sodus and 5.25 miles west of the intersection of NY 89 and NY 104 near Wolcott, from NY 104, turn north onto CR 254/Lake Bluff Road. CR 254/Lake Bluff Road becomes Garner Road. Continue north along Garner Road, and stay right at the sharp turn east (right), at 5.5 miles. Shortly after this turn, the main parking area for Chimney Bluffs State Park will be on your left. To reach the East Bay Road parking area, continue 0.9 mile along Garner Road. Turn left onto East Bay Road. The parking area is another 0.9 mile ahead on the left.

3

Beaver Lake
Nature Center

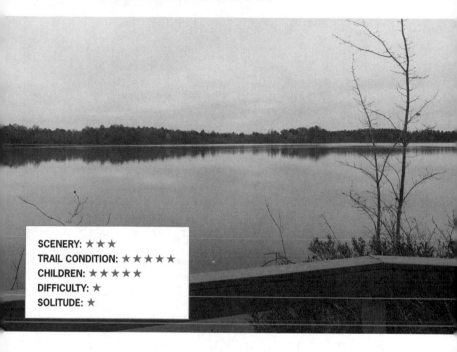

SCENERY: ★ ★ ★
TRAIL CONDITION: ★ ★ ★ ★ ★
CHILDREN: ★ ★ ★ ★ ★
DIFFICULTY: ★
SOLITUDE: ★

GPS TRAILHEAD COORDINATES: (Lake Loop) N43° 10.855'   W76° 24.127'

DISTANCE & CONFIGURATION: 3.0-mile Lake Loop; 1.5-mile Three Meadows Loop; 1.4-mile Deep Woods Loop. 5.9 miles total, with multiple smaller loops and side trips available.

HIKING TIME: 2.5 hours for all three loops described

HIGHLIGHTS: Pristine lake, boardwalks, nature center

ELEVATION: 536' at Lake Loop trailhead, with no significant change in elevation

ACCESS: Daily, 7:30 a.m.–sunset; closed Thanksgiving and December 25; $4 vehicle access fee

MAPS: onondagacountyparks.com/beaver-lake-nature-center; also available at nature center

FACILITIES: Restrooms, nature center, arboretum

WHEELCHAIR ACCESS: Limited to special programs

COMMENTS: No dogs allowed. Pay the entrance fee at the nature center, where you will receive the necessary exit ticket to get past the barrier gate.

CONTACTS: Beaver Lake Nature Center, 315-638-2519, onondagacountyparks.com /beaver-lake-nature-center

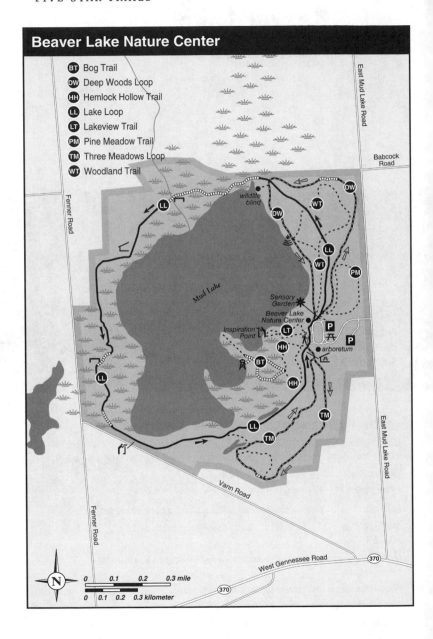

Beaver Lake Nature Center

- BT   Bog Trail
- DW   Deep Woods Loop
- HH   Hemlock Hollow Trail
- LL   Lake Loop
- LT   Lakeview Trail
- PM   Pine Meadow Trail
- TM   Three Meadows Loop
- WT   Woodland Trail

Overview

Just northwest of Syracuse, Beaver Lake Nature Center is an excellent excursion for families or anyone who simply wants to enjoy a serene lakeside stroll. The lake trail is popular among runners, while the short loops near the nature center are favorites for families with children and toddlers alike.

Route Details

The trails here are in excellent condition; some sections are mulched, providing a soft cushion underfoot, while the sections traversing wetlands have boardwalks to minimize environmental impacts. The park keeps a heavy emphasis on education and engagement with the public. You can certainly explore the park on your own, as I did, but you may be interested in participating in the more than 400 programs and events offered annually. These programs include workshops and lectures that focus on natural history, storytelling, nature-inspired art, and environmental conservation. The staff and associated parties also offer additional hands-on programs and activities, such as introduction to snowshoeing, GPS scavenger hunts, and canoe tours. I happened to visit the park around Halloween during one of its more popular events, Enchanted Beaver Lake, which featured 400-plus jack-o-lanterns distributed along the shorter trails to illuminate them. According to staff, the event had been completely sold out for all the dates, October 25–28. For your visit, upcoming events are available to download on the park's website. The trails described below are the three largest loops: Lake Loop (3 miles), Three Meadows Loop (1.5 miles), and Deep Woods Loop (1.4 miles), all of which can be combined to create a 5.9-mile trip.

Lake Loop (3 miles)

Begin this trail just past the Sensory Garden, beneath a handsome sign marking the trail beginning; similar signs mark the other trails too. The initial leg of the loop weaves through a hardwood forest and is intersected a few times by neighboring trails, the Woodland Trail and Deep Woods Trail (described later on). Continue straight, northward, through each of these intersections along a heavily mulched trail. The trail is very easygoing, and you soon leave behind this cluster of trails and reach the first section of boardwalk. The trail is now heading westward and, for the next roughly 0.5 mile, weaves its way through a wetland on the north shore of Mud Lake. The wide boardwalk lets you traverse some impassable and inaccessible habitats that provide excellent wildlife viewing as well as some scenic vistas of the lake. The boardwalk continues along much of the northern shore and crosses Mud Lake inlet at 0.9 mile and ends shortly afterward, roughly one-third around the circuit. The trail winds its way back toward the lakeshore, and you soon come upon a trail shelter to your left. Near the shelter, paths down to the shoreline provide excellent panoramic views of the lake. After heading westward briefly, you begin to near the park's boundary just as the trail bends to the left, southward. The next 0.3 mile is an easy jaunt, and you soon reach an elevated boardwalk, approximately 1.7 miles ahead. Mud Lake's outlet weaves through this area, and just before you reach the end of the boardwalk section, a small viewing platform and bench provide seating above a cattail marsh. You will cross the Mud Lake outlet again, over a short bridge and then a boardwalk, just before the trail begins to head eastward. As you come into view of a neighboring road (Vann Road) around the 2-mile mark, you will notice an observation tower that includes a telescope.

As you make your way along the southern shore, the trail follows a more elevated path along the lake. Approximately 2.3 miles in, you intersect a short spur trail to Three Meadows Loop, with signage indicating as much. You can follow this trail back if you would like to add some ecological variety to your trip, or add this loop after completing the Lake Loop. At 2.5 miles you reach a small pond and have only 0.5 mile left to reach the end of the loop. The loop essentially concludes at a pavilion that neighbors an open lawn.

From here you can add Three Meadows Loop or Deep Woods Loop, or conclude your trip.

Three Meadows Loop (1.5 miles)

This short loop adds a brief moment of solitude to your trip, while also allowing you to experience a different type of environment. The Lake Loop and other loops near the nature center seem to be more popular, and I encountered people on those trails every 10 minutes or so. On the other hand, on this loop I not only didn't see another person but I couldn't even hear anyone, even though this was a very busy weekend at the park. To begin the loop, head past the pavilion and then south toward the arboretum. The Three Meadows trail begins with a brief stint through a stand of white pines, passes through an open lawn and back into a stand of pines, and then weaves through mature hardwoods. By now you might begin to wonder where the meadows are, but less than 0.5 mile in, the trail transitions from forest to field. Birch trees dot this first section of open field. Benches are scattered along this loop, as they are along all the trails, and you can't help but feel that, if you sit for a brief while, something is sure to pass through. The area is riddled with transition zones, niches between two ecological habitats. These boundary areas share characteristics with each habitat and are often active areas for wildlife. No doubt you are likely to be rewarded with some wildlife views here if you slow your pace or even stop and observe. At roughly 0.6 mile, you pass the spur trail that connects to Lake Loop. Past the spur, the trail heads eastward, winding through fields much of the way. You reenter the forest near its conclusion and shortly after encounter the open lawn by the pavilion.

Deep Woods Loop (1.4 miles)

The Deep Woods Loop is yet another opportunity to find some seclusion in the busy park, especially around the eastern and northern portions. Much of the ecology is similar to the forest that surrounds the lake, with the exception of the eastern portion, which consists of dense conifers. My recommended routing for the loop is to begin near the Pine Meadow Trailhead and conclude near the visitor center.

The trail begins by passing between the Pine Meadow Trail, to your right, and the Lake Loop, to your left, but you soon pass out of sight of these trails. The setting takes on a primeval feel as the dense conifers close in around you. However, this setting is brief and the typical hardwood forest emerges again as you cross a brief boardwalk section, 0.4 mile in. At approximately 0.75 mile, you intersect the Lake Loop and shortly after reach a short spur to your right that leads to a wildlife blind beside Mud Lake. From this point, the trail weaves its way along the lakeshore back to the nature center, and there are benches at a few excellent spots to view the lake. You will even pass by the park's amphitheater and boat rental. For a deep woods route, this offers a great deal of lakeside strolling, and you might want to consider substituting this section for the beginning or end of a circuit around the lake.

Directions

From the end of I-690, continue on NY 690 North for 5.7 miles and take Exit NY 31 West/NY 370/West Gennessee Road. Turn right onto NY 31 West/NY 370/West Gennessee Road. Turn right on CR 180/East Mud Lake Road at 1.8 miles. Follow this road 0.8 mile, and the park entrance is on your left.

Howland Island

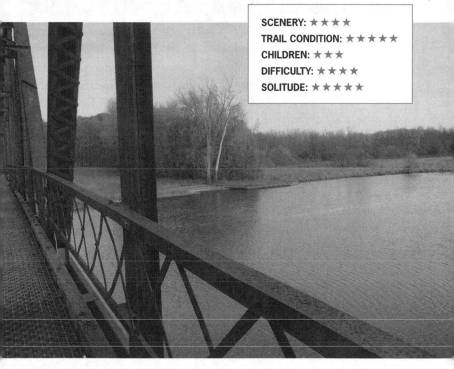

SCENERY: ★ ★ ★ ★
TRAIL CONDITION: ★ ★ ★ ★ ★
CHILDREN: ★ ★ ★
DIFFICULTY: ★ ★ ★ ★
SOLITUDE: ★ ★ ★ ★ ★

GPS TRAILHEAD COORDINATES: (parking area on Howland Island Road) N43° 04.001'
W76° 40.020'

DISTANCE & CONFIGURATION: 5.75-mile loop

HIKING TIME: 2–3 hours

HIGHLIGHTS: Isolated ponds, vast wetlands, prime wildlife viewing

ELEVATION: 380' at trailhead, with no significant change in elevation

ACCESS: Open 24/7; no fees or permits required

MAPS: Area map: **dec.ny.gov/outdoor/27393.html**; also available at visitor center

FACILITIES: None

WHEELCHAIR ACCESS: No

COMMENTS: To see the most wildlife, plan your trip during the spring and fall migrations.
This is a popular spot for duck hunting, so be mindful if you visit during the hunting season
(typically mid-October–early January). Equestrians share the trail.

CONTACTS: NYSDEC Region 8 Headquarters, 585-226-2466, **dec.ny.gov/outdoor
/31112.html**

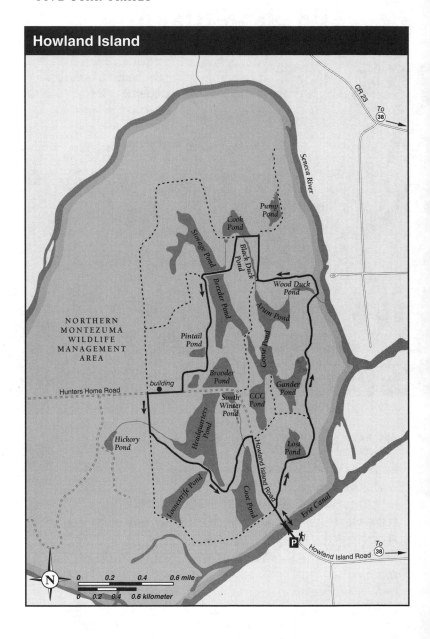

Howland Island

Seneca River

CR 23

To 38

Pump Pond

Cook Pond

Storage Pond

Black Duck Pond

Wood Duck Pond

Breeder Pond

Arum Pond

Goose Pond

NORTHERN MONTEZUMA WILDLIFE MANAGEMENT AREA

Pintail Pond

Brooder Pond

Gander Pond

building

Hunters Home Road

South Winter Pond

CCC Pond

Headquarters Pond

Hickory Pond

Lost Pond

Howland Island Road

Loosestrife Pond

Coot Pond

Erie Canal

P

To 38

Howland Island Road

N

| 0 | 0.2 | 0.4 | 0.6 mile |
| 0 | 0.2 | 0.4 | 0.6 kilometer |

Overview

Along the northern edge of the Finger Lakes is a vast network of wild-life refuges primarily made up of the 7,068-acre federal Montezuma National Wildlife Refuge (described below) and the 7,700-acre state-run Northern Montezuma Wildlife Management Area, which is further subdivided into the South Butler, Savannah, and Howland Island Units. Encompassing 3,100 acres, Howland Island is not exactly how you would picture an island, but indeed it is surrounded by the Seneca River on the east, north, and west, while the "new" Erie Canal forms its southern boundary. But the image of an island is somewhat misleading, as most of the time it seems that there is more water on the island than surrounding it. Most of the area is marshland, with roughly 300 acres of man-made ponds/impoundments that provide habitat for more than 220 bird species, 108 of which are considered local breeders. The trail system is a network of access roads that circle and weave through the numerous ponds and wetlands.

Route Details

From the parking area beside Howland Island Road, head over the steel trestle bridge. The island bridge extends high above the Erie Canal with multiple panoramic views. On the right side of the opposing shore is a boat landing site that provides boat access to the island. The Department of Environmental Conservation (DEC) maintains several public boat launch sites nearby; the closest are to the north on the Seneca River. A list of DEC boat launches specific to the Northern Montezuma Wildlife Management Area is available at **dec.ny.gov/docs/fish _marine_pdf/montsencaybls.pdf.**

Soon after you reach the island shore, you will come to a four-way intersection. To the left is the Eagle Hill Trail (not featured in the loop described), straight ahead is the central road and the return leg of the trip, and to the right is the beginning of the loop heading northeast to Lost Pond. A little over 0.3 mile down the gravel road, Lost Pond lies awash in cattails from shore to shore. Take your pictures of this

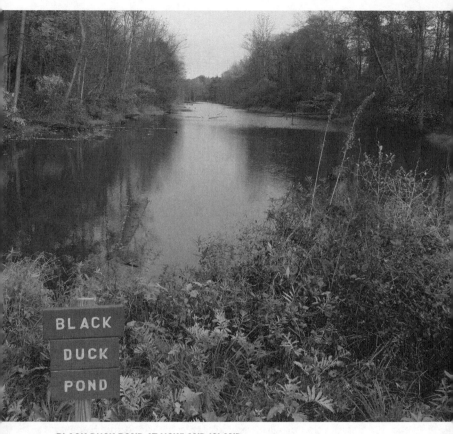

BLACK DUCK POND AT HOWLAND ISLAND

pond as you pass along its southern berm, because once you reach the eastern edge, thick brush masks the pond from view.

At 0.8 mile you reach a fork in the trail. To the left is a brief side trip to Gander Pond, the eastern shore of CCC Pond, and the southern tip of Goose Pond. There used to be a path that allowed hikers to explore an interior route through these ponds, but the bridge/berm dividing Goose and Gander Ponds has been removed. It is roughly 0.5 mile to the dead-end, so if you choose to include this diversion in the trip, it will add 1 mile to the overall hike length. Along this side trip, views of CCC Pond are mostly obscured by the surrounding understory, but the meeting point of Goose Pond and Gander Pond is quite scenic; keep an eye out for the beaver lodge.

Back on the main loop, continue straight at the fork for 0.25 mile, when you arrive at an opening in the forest that provides sprawling views of Gander Pond. Just ahead, you reach the north tip of the pond and a T-intersection. To the left are an open field and a road that was the old route between the ponds, while the outer loop and path forward lie to the right.

In about 0.25 mile, or 1.5 miles overall, you will reach the eastern tip of Wood Duck Pond, with the Seneca River just visible off to the right. The trail swings around to the north shore of Wood Duck Pond and begins a gentle 0.25-mile climb to an open hilltop. Follow the field down to the bottom of the drumlin, where there is another trail intersection. To the left are Arum Pond and the central road that leads back to Goose and CCC Ponds. To the right is a road that follows Black Duck Pond almost due north. Turn right and travel 0.3 mile to where a field opens up on your left and you soon reach another intersection. The road continues briefly north and then east to Pump Pond, while our route goes downhill and to the left toward the berm between Black Duck and Cook Ponds, at 2.3 miles. Once across the berm, head up the gravel road and reach yet another intersection. Going straight, or westward, will take you on a much longer route around the perimeter of the management area. This route leads to the northern tip of Storage Pond, but after that offers little else related to the ponds. So instead, turn to your left and south, where a road takes you alongside Breeder Pond, Pintail Pond, and Brooder Pond, and provides perhaps the most scenic portion of the trip.

The road heads nearly due south, and as it begins to make a brief swing westward, the forest disappears and a panorama of open water and fields surrounds you. Breeder Pond sprawls out to the south while Storage Pond fills the view to the north as the road veers westward. Watch closely for the beaver lodge nestled in the middle of Storage Pond. At the end of the berm between the two ponds, you reach the midway point along the loop and a sharp turn south through a hedgerow. Along the next 0.25 mile, the trail stays almost entirely in the open, with Breeder Pond filling the landscape to your left and an agricultural field on your right. These fields are used to grow food for wildlife, which further enhances the refuge's attraction for migratory birds. After a short zigzag through a tiny copse of woods, you will pass Pintail Pond on your right, at 3.3 miles. Shortly after, the road turns westward just around a tiny stand of pine trees and then swings south again before intersecting the main access road. To the left, east, is the main road that first crosses between Brooder Pond and Headquarters Pond, and then swings south toward the trestle bridge. You could return this way, effectively shortening your trip by 0.75 mile, but to take in even more of the area, I recommend turning right so you can circumnavigate Headquarters Pond and take in brief views of Loosestrife and Coot Ponds as well.

Head due west about 0.25 mile, past the metal building on the right, to a four-way road intersection. Turn left, south, and follow the gravel road to a fork, at 4.1 miles overall. If you travel straight ahead, the gravel road will swing around the southern tips of Loosestrife and Coot Ponds and eventually reach the four-way intersection first encountered after the trestle bridge crossing. The route I chose, however, follows the grassy road along the left side of the fork. Here tall grasses fill the landscape, but they soon give way to open waters at the 4.5-mile point, where a berm between Loosestrife and Headquarters Ponds is reached. The road swings south and then arrives at another fork. Bear left onto the more developed road and follow it southeast a short way to where the road turns sharply left, heading northeast. Roughly 0.3 mile farther, descend to the southern tip of South Winter Pond, where the road turns east and then reconnects with the main road, at just over 5 miles overall. Turn right on the main road to head back to the trestle bridge, 0.75 mile ahead to the south, for an overall trip length of 5.75 miles (6.75 miles if you added the side trip to Goose Pond). As you head south, keep an eye open for a large boulder with a memorial plaque on the left. The plaque is located at the site of the original Civilian Conservation

Corps camp used to help build the complex, which soon after was briefly repurposed as a German prisoner of war camp.

Nearby Attractions

Though the Montezuma National Wildlife Refuge is open during daylight hours seven days a week, most visitors will choose to take the 3.5-mile wildlife drive. The drive opens in April and closes when snow and ice prevent safe travel through the complex (generally when the visitor center is closed). The drive weaves through different habitats and alongside different pools, with a self-guided phone tour that complements the experience. The visitor center (315-568-5987) also features a short hiking trail and is one place where actual maps of the Northern Montezuma Wildlife Management Area can be found. Ideal times to visit are during the spring and fall migrations. Summer activities include watching local birds nesting and brood-rearing, while during the winter you can cross-country ski or snowshoe the wildlife drive.

Directions

From I-90, take Exit 40 (NY 34/Weedsport/Auburn). Turn right on NY 34 South, and then turn right on NY 31 West/Erie Drive after 0.8 mile. After 3.9 miles, stay right to remain on NY 31/Rochester Street. Turn right on NY 38 North after 0.4 mile. Follow NY 38 North for 1.8 miles, and turn left onto CR 139/Howland Island Road. Follow CR 139/Howland Island Road 1.8 miles to the large pulloff beside the road just in front of the steel bridge.

East (Hikes 5–15)

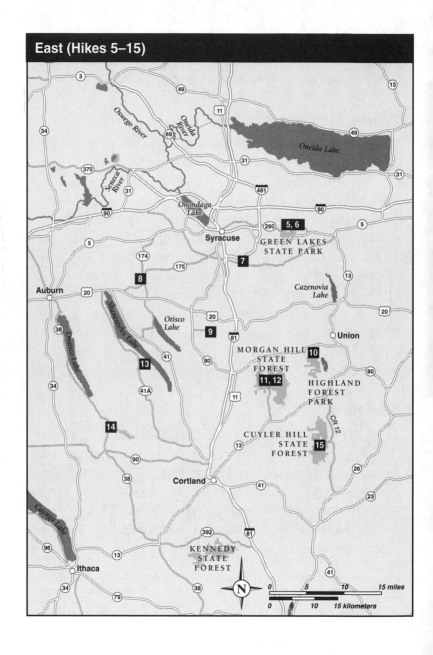

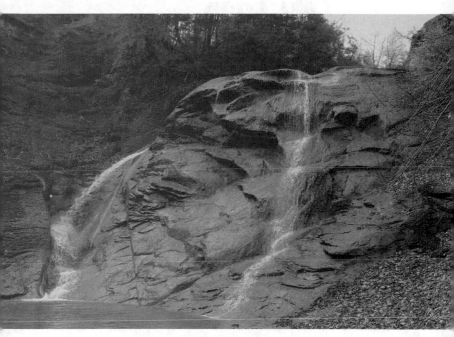

TRAIL 9 GREAT FALLS AT RATTLESNAKE GULF & ADAMS EDEN CAMP
see page 83

5 Green Lakes State Park: Lake Loop

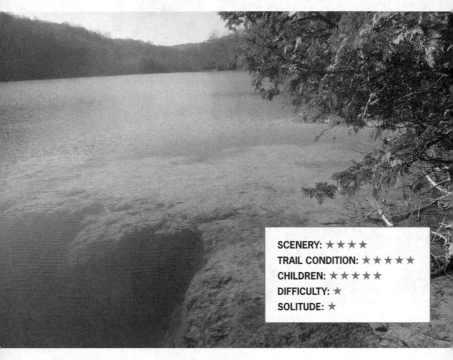

SCENERY: ★ ★ ★ ★
TRAIL CONDITION: ★ ★ ★ ★ ★
CHILDREN: ★ ★ ★ ★ ★
DIFFICULTY: ★
SOLITUDE: ★

GPS TRAILHEAD COORDINATES: (north park entrance) N43° 03.586′   W75° 58.280′
(Lake Loop trailhead) N43° 03.419′   W75° 57.876′

DISTANCE & CONFIGURATION: 3.0-mile loop

HIKING TIME: 1–1.5 hours

HIGHLIGHTS: Meromictic lakes, swimming beach

ELEVATION: 390′ at trailhead, with no significant rise

ACCESS: Daily, sunrise–sunset; $8 vehicle entrance fee

MAPS: nysparks.com/parks/172/maps.aspx; also available on-site

FACILITIES: Restrooms, concessions, swimming area, picnic area, golf course, boat rental, campground

WHEELCHAIR ACCESS: Yes

COMMENTS: The trail around the lake is very popular all year long for walkers, family outings, and runners. Dogs are allowed on leash but not in the bathing area. No swimming outside designated areas.

CONTACTS: Green Lakes State Park, 315-637-6111, nysparks.com/parks/172 /details.aspx

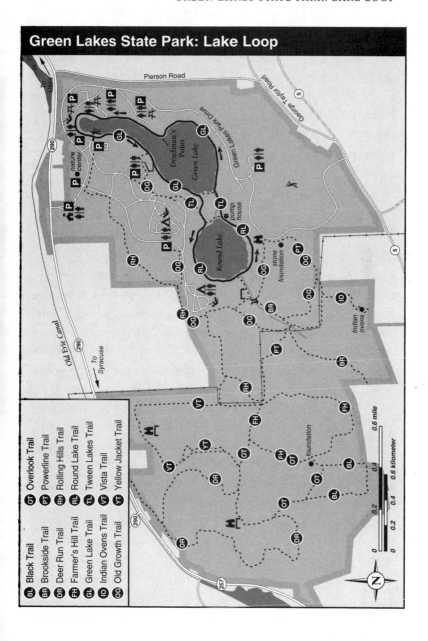

Green Lakes State Park: Lake Loop

Overview

The loop around Green and Round Lakes is one of the flattest and easiest trails featured in the book. Often crowded and certainly busy any time of the year, this park won't provide privacy (for that, add the Farmer's Hill loop featured on page 64). So why would a crowded and easy stroll be included in a hiking book? Simply put, the rare nature of these lakes makes them a must-see for anyone exploring the region. These lakes offer a literal and illustrative window into the natural forces that shaped the present-day landscape.

Route Details

The route around both Green and Round Lakes is well developed and one of the main reasons the park is so popular with walkers and runners. But the other reason is the unusual appearance and peculiar nature of these pristine lakes (more on that later). The path around the lakes can be explored in any direction; indeed it would be hard to get lost along the lake loops, but I recommend a counterclockwise direction so that you save some of Green Lake's more complex and interesting reef features for near the end.

The sprawling parking area encompasses the northern edge of the lake, so your starting point will actually vary. For simplicity's sake, keep the lake on your left and navigate past the swimming area along the western shore to where the path plunges into a cedar grove; mileage will be given from this point. A short way ahead, you pass stairs that lead up to the Pine Woods Camping Area (for a description of the campground, see *Best Tent Camping: New York State*).

Continue straight along this sinuous bay to where the lake begins to broaden. As you progress, the banks of the lake drop off precipitously into unfathomable greenish depths below. Indeed there seems to be a murky barrier between the crystal-clear water near the surface and something below. The juxtaposition is not an illusion, but a real transition between two distinct layers of water and the source of the park's name and allure.

Both Green and Round Lakes are meromictic lakes—lakes whose top and bottom layers do not intermix. They are a rare form of lake and extraordinarily so in temperate climates. In shallow lakes, water intermixes frequently through turbidity, but in deep lakes the intermixing of surface and deeper water occurs mostly because of temperature differentials from the changing of seasons. For instance, in the fall as surface water cools, it becomes denser and sinks, while the relatively warmer water from the depths rises to the surface. However, this seasonal intermixing does not occur here. Why? Partly it is a function of the lakes' depth-to-surface ratio; partly it is a function of the sheltering gorge walls that limit the amount of change in surface temperature and mixing due to wind. But the meromictic nature of these lakes also derives from their atypical water chemistry. The groundwater that supplies the lake is heavily laden with minerals and salts, mostly calcium carbonate from the surrounding limestone. This denser, briny water adds yet another barrier to the waters intermixing. It is the high concentration of calcium carbonate in the water that imbues Green Lake with its bluish-green tint and gives the park its name.

The boundary between the two water types is called a chemocline and occurs roughly at 60 feet below the surface. At the chemocline, an interesting array of bacteria and algae exist, including a purple sulfur bacteria that creates a pink band. Below this boundary, the water is anoxic (devoid of oxygen) and little life exists. As such, the detritus of millennia remains undisturbed by decomposition or organisms, and layer upon layer of sediment forms a virtual record of the environment for thousands of years. So what lies beyond the murky barrier is surprisingly more complex than you might think.

As you near the southern end of the lake, you reach the first of two crossover trails; bear right onto the first crossover trail. As you crest a small hill, you intersect a road that leads back to the campgrounds on your right. Bear left and down a slight incline to Round Lake, and turn right to circumnavigate the lake in the counterclockwise direction. Though Round Lake is very similar to Green Lake, it

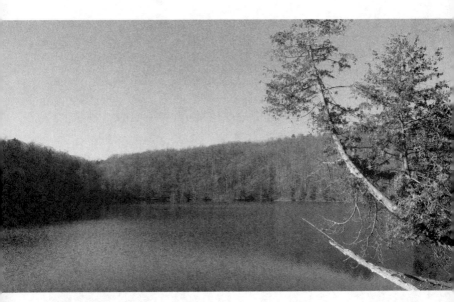

GREEN LAKE

has a smaller diameter and feels more hemmed in by the surrounding gorge walls. In this setting, contemplating how these lakes were formed takes on a starker contrast.

As is the case with many of the other trails featured in this book, massive glaciers sculpted the landscape at Green Lakes State Park as well. While the ice bulldozed, scoured, and flattened the surrounding landscape, the transformation here was a bit different. As the ice receded northward, meltwater poured over the trailing edge of the ice. These glacial waterfalls dug into the soft limestone, gouging out deep plunge pools, far deeper than any present-day water source could create. Surrounding Round Lake, which is 180 feet deep, are 150-foot-high gorge walls; Green Lake is 195 feet deep. Dig through the sediment that has accumulated at the bottom of the lake, and the actual lake depth may be another 150 feet. Now imagine the waterfall that digs through nearly 500 feet of rock and think of the scale of the glaciers, and their influence becomes daunting. To see a smaller-scale version of this process in action, visit Buttermilk Falls (page 157 or 164) or Watkins Glen (page 194).

Near the halfway point and the southwest end of Round Lake, a steep trail comes down to the lake on the right. Up this trail are the more recent additions to the park and some unique aspects that can be explored further in the Farmer's Hill loop described on page 64. Continue around the south shore of Round Lake, and take the second crossover trail to return to Green Lake and follow its southern shore back to the swimming area.

At 2.33 miles, you pass by Deadman's Point, an oddly whitish peninsula akin to a coral reef that extends southwest into the lake. Though similar protrusions are visible elsewhere around the lake, the shore leading up to and around this point is the most stunning. How this marl reef is formed is yet another of the peculiar characteristics of the lake. More than half of the water that feeds the lake is from groundwater, which, as stated earlier, is laden with calcium carbonate. Eventually these salts precipitate from the water, and the lake undergoes an annual "whiting" as the solidified minerals add new layers to fallen trees and bulbous outcrops. Millennia of precipitate accumulation have created reefs and an almost primordial scene along the outcrop. From Deadman's Point, it's another 0.6 mile to the swimming area, concessions, and parking area, for a total loop length of 3 miles (8 miles if you added the Farmer's Hill loop to your trip).

Directions

From I-481, take Exit 3E (East Genesee Street/NY 5E) toward Fayetteville. Head east on East Genesee Street/NY 5 about 1 mile and stay left at the fork to remain on East Genesee Street/NY 5. Continue 2 miles and turn left on North Manlius Street/NY 257. At 1.8 miles, North Manlius Street/NY 257 becomes Green Lakes Road/NY 290. Continue along Green Lakes Road/NY 290 for 1.6 miles, and the park entrance will be on the right.

Green Lakes State Park: Farmer's Hill

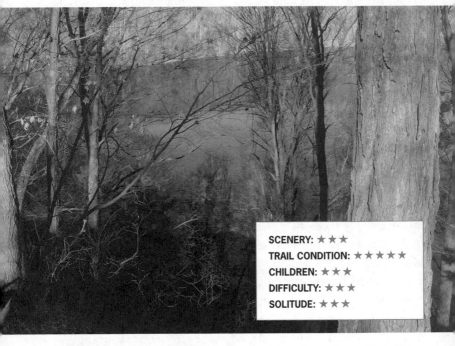

SCENERY: ★ ★ ★
TRAIL CONDITION: ★ ★ ★ ★ ★
CHILDREN: ★ ★ ★
DIFFICULTY: ★ ★ ★
SOLITUDE: ★ ★ ★

GPS TRAILHEAD COORDINATES: (north park entrance) N43° 03.586' W75° 58.280'
(Lake Loop trailhead) N43° 03.419' W75° 57.876'
(Beginning at Round Lake) N43° 02.805' W75° 58.650'

DISTANCE & CONFIGURATION: 4.9-mile loop; 7.9-mile figure eight if combined
with Lake Loop

HIKING TIME: 1.5–2 hours along loop; 2.5–3.5 hours combined with Lake Loop

HIGHLIGHTS: Old-growth forests, open fields, panoramic views

ELEVATION: 420' at trail beginning along Round Lake; 710' at highest point along loop

ACCESS: Daily, sunrise–sunset; $8 vehicle entrance fee

MAPS: nysparks.com/parks/172/maps.aspx; also available on-site

FACILITIES: Restrooms, concessions, swimming area, picnic area, golf course, boat rental,
campground

WHEELCHAIR ACCESS: No

COMMENTS: The trail network through old-growth forests and open fields is shared with
bikers. Dogs are allowed on leash but not allowed in the bathing area.

CONTACTS: Green Lakes State Park, 315-637-6111, nysparks.com/parks/172
/details.aspx

Overview

Of this park's 1,955 acres, more than half of the acreage lies above and beyond the lakes. Yet many of the visitors to Green Lakes State Park don't realize that the park extends far beyond the lakeside trails—which is unfortunate, for these visitors miss out on some truly distinctive aspects of the park, most notably the extensive old-growth forest surrounding Round Lake. But, fortunately for you, much of the trails in the upper part of the parks will be relatively uncrowded. There still are many runners, bikers, and occasional hikers that venture up into the open fields and old-growth forest, but nothing like the crowds that stroll around the lakes.

Route Details

From the intersection of the Brookside Trail at the southwest end of Round Lake, head up the short 100-foot climb and reach a bench near a fork in the trail. Straight ahead are a small bridge and the conclusion of the loop, but for now turn right and head uphill, following the Old Growth Trail, marked in orange. Along the climb, 100 feet over 0.25 mile, you intersect another section of the Old Growth Trail network on the left; continue ascending along the right-hand path to the intersection with the yellow Rolling Hills Trail. To the right is the Rolling Hills Camping Area, as well as the continuation of the Old Growth Trail that passes by the Pine Woods Camping Area and eventually goes back to the main parking area, roughly 1 mile to the northeast. Turn left and follow the yellow trail markers through the forest 0.4 mile to the intersection with the green Vista Trail. Bear right on the Vista Trail and proceed to where the trail leaves the forest and enters into open fields below power lines, approximately 1 mile from the start at Round Lake. Turn right and follow the hedgerow almost due north a little over 0.3 mile until a side path leads off to the right. Turn left to stay on the Vista Trail, and soon a panoramic view to the north opens where Oneida Lake sprawls across the horizon.

Green Lakes State Park: Farmer's Hill

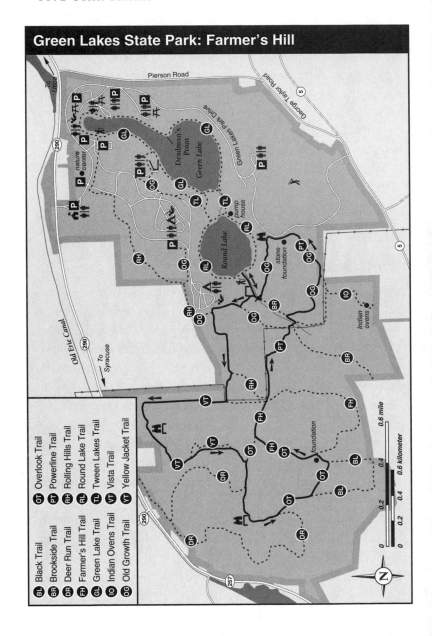

Legend:

- BL Black Trail
- BR Brookside Trail
- DR Deer Run Trail
- FH Farmer's Hill Trail
- GL Green Lake Trail
- IO Indian Ovens Trail
- OG Old Growth Trail
- OT Overlook Trail
- PT Powerline Trail
- RH Rolling Hills Trail
- RL Round Lake Trail
- TL Tween Lakes Trail
- VT Vista Trail
- YT Yellow Jacket Trail

Oneida Lake, 21 miles long and 5 miles wide, has some of the characteristics of a finger lake; it's long and narrow but averages only 22 feet deep and runs east to west. Its formation was not the deep scouring of an ancient river valley as found in other finger lakes, nor was Oneida scooped out as a plunge pool like the pothole lakes Round, Green, and Glacier (see the Clark Reservation trail described on page 70). Nevertheless it too was shaped and formed by the receding glaciers, though its creation was more similar to that of the Great Lakes than the Finger Lakes.

Head west along the mown trail for about 0.3 mile until the trail turns sharply left and crosses a wooded ravine. Intersect the Yellow Jacket Trail on the left shortly after. This short spur explores the ravine a brief way and should not be confused with Deer Run Trail, also marked in yellow and encountered farther ahead. Continue straight along the green trail, following the ravine briefly south before intersecting with the red Overlook Trail. The yellow, green, and red trails all combine as you bear right and head west. A short way ahead, the Deer Run loop departs on the right; adding this longer yellow loop would extend your trip by roughly 1.5 miles. Continue straight along the multicolored trail and be rewarded with a sprawling view of communities to the west as the trail swings to the left. Continue south, past the re-intersection with the Deer Run Trail, and then head east briefly until

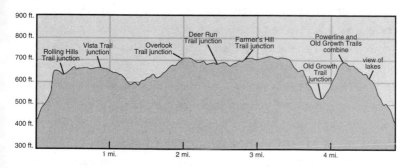

you intersect an old gravel road. To your left are the remains of a barn foundation, once part of a cluster of farm buildings that occupied this hilltop. When I was boy, the house, silo, barn, and livestock pens still stood, but all that remains today are these stones and a few scraggly trees slightly at odds with the open fields. Head north along the road about 0.5 mile, and turn right at the intersection toward the overhead power lines. Follow the power lines down the hill, marked with white blazes. The Rolling Hills Trail soon departs on the left, heading into the forest. A short way ahead along the power lines, the trail diverts to the right and plunges back into the forest.

After a meandering descent of 100 feet over 0.25 mile, the trail reconnects with the power lines and briefly follows them east, past the blue-marked Brookside Trail on the right, and then reaches a fork. The white trail continues to follow the power lines, while the orange Old Growth Trail turns left back into the woods. Follow the latter, and soon after you reenter the forest, the orange trail will turn right and head uphill. Follow this long climb, 150 feet over 0.3 mile, and again intersect the white trail just as the back of a neighborhood and a house come into view. Stay left and follow the orange trail to an intersection with a road and service area. Bear left and follow the road a short way while looking for the orange-marked trail heading back into the woods on the left side of the road.

Shortly after reentering the forest, intersect the white golf course crossover trail. Though I don't recommend heading over to the golf course (except perhaps in winter for excellent skiing and snowshoeing), there is an excellent sight to take in a very short way down this trail, especially during the fall and winter. As you crest a small knoll, you'll gain a sprawling view of Round Lake and the tip of Green Lake glimpsed through the canopy of trees that line the rim and basin walls. From here you have a new perspective of the scale of the waterfall that carved these lakes.

Return to the orange trail and begin to descend back to the bench near the start of the loop. If you had not noticed the amazing girth of some trees within this forest, you are sure to now. Fifty-nine acres of forest surrounding Round Lake are designated as old-growth forest, a rare thing in New York State. Old-growth forests are characterized by multilayered canopies, large-diameter trees, broad forest gaps from individual tree falls, and large woody debris across the forest floor. As you can imagine, old-growth forests take shape over time, 150–500 years minimum. Most of New York's forests were cut down as the region was colonized and converted to agriculture. Over the past century the forest began to rebound, but forestry practices often advocated cutting larger diameter trees for their economic value, and few forest giants were allowed to grow and re-create the old-growth forest that once covered the Northeast. But here there are trees 4 feet in diameter, and some are estimated to be more than 350 years old. The unusual nature of the lakes and the old-growth forest here are some of the reasons that Round Lake was designated as a National Natural Landmark in 1973.

After the orange trail reconnects with the blue, the two cross a shallow stream over a wooden bridge and reach the top of the trail down to the meromictic lakes. From here it's another 1.75 miles back to the swimming area and parking area, for an overall trip length of 7.9 miles.

Directions

From I-481, take Exit 3E (East Genesee Street/NY 5E) toward Fayetteville. Head east on East Genesee Street/NY 5 for about 1 mile and stay left at the fork to remain on East Genesee Street/NY 5. Continue 2 miles and turn left on North Manlius Street/NY 257. At 1.8 miles, North Manlius Street/NY 257 becomes Green Lakes Road/NY 290. Continue along Green Lakes Road/NY 290 for 1.6 miles, and the park entrance will be on the right.

Clark Reservation
State Park

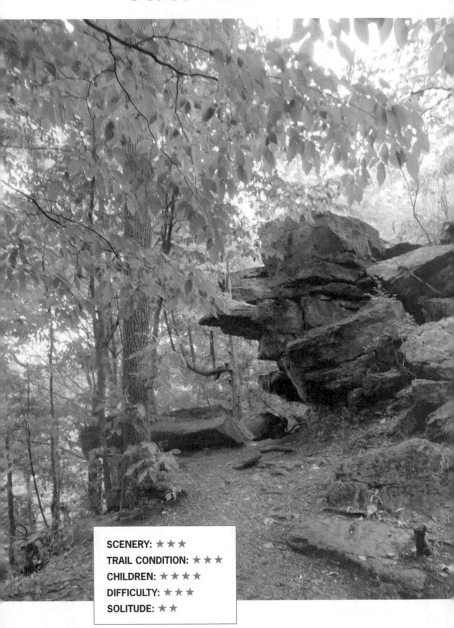

SCENERY: ★ ★ ★
TRAIL CONDITION: ★ ★ ★
CHILDREN: ★ ★ ★ ★
DIFFICULTY: ★ ★ ★
SOLITUDE: ★ ★

GPS TRAILHEAD COORDINATES: (parking area) N42° 59.686'   W76° 05.696'

DISTANCE & CONFIGURATION: 1.0-mile Lower Lake Loop; 2.25-mile Upper Rim Loop

HIKING TIME: 1–2 hours

HIGHLIGHTS: Meromictic lake, steep cliffs, vistas

ELEVATION: 730' in parking area; 590' at lowest point along Lower Lake Loop

ACCESS: Daily, sunrise–sunset; $4 vehicle entrance fee

MAPS: nysparks.com/parks/126/maps.aspx; also available at entrance booth

FACILITIES: Restrooms, playground, nature center, picnic shelters

WHEELCHAIR ACCESS: No

COMMENTS: The stairs down to Glacier Lake and the trail along the rim are closed during the winter. Sections of the trail are shared with mountain bikers.

CONTACTS: Clark Reservation State Park, 315-492-1590, **nysparks.com/parks/126 /details.aspx**

Overview

If you feel that the trails around Green Lakes State Park are too developed and you want to explore something with a wilder feel, then the trails at Clark Reservation might just hit the spot. The park also features a meromictic lake, but unlike the routes of its brethren, Green and Round Lakes, the path around Glacier Lake is rough and rocky, so you will find far fewer hikers/runners. The trails are still popular and the park is fairly small, at 325 acres, so don't expect solitude. But the trails are more rugged and offer a change of pace from other state park hikes. Indeed, with the varied terrain and different niches encountered along the network of trails here, it's hard to believe the park is so small.

Route Details

A multitude of routes of varying lengths are available along this network of trails, and I've divided the trail into two sections: the Upper Rim Loop, 2.25 miles, and the Lower Lake Loop, 1 mile. The Upper Rim Loop follows many small sections of the various trails interwoven in the upper section of the park. Many alternative routes could be explored, but I've chosen a hike that takes in some of what each trail has to offer. I encourage you to explore the options for yourself,

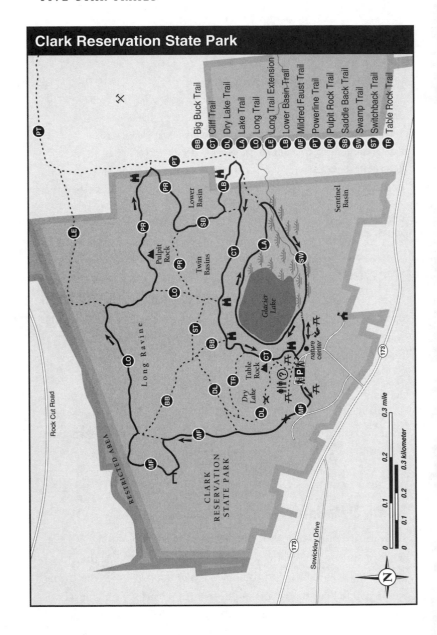

Clark Reservation State Park

BB Big Buck Trail
CT Cliff Trail
DL Dry Lake Trail
LA Lake Trail
LO Long Trail
LE Long Trail Extension
LB Lower Basin Trail
MF Mildred Faust Trail
PT Powerline Trail
PR Pulpit Rock Trail
SB Saddle Back Trail
SW Swamp Trail
ST Switchback Trail
TR Table Rock Trail

as there is lots to discover, especially for aspiring naturalists (see below). The Lower Lake Loop is simply a circumnavigation of Glacier Lake. The two loops can be hiked independently or combined by utilizing the crossover trail near the eastern end of the lake. Both are short loops, so I recommend hiking them both.

Upper Rim Loop

The Upper Rim Loop begins along the Mildred Faust Trail, located on the western end of the parking area. You first pass through some play and administration areas, but will soon leave them behind as the trail swings northward after crossing a short bridge. Continue straight past the first trail junction, a crossover trail that connects to the interior of the upper loop section. At the second trail junction you can continue straight to directly access the Long Trail or bear left and continue on the Mildred Faust Trail along a short loop. The loop is uneventful and passes by many of the unofficial trails scattered along the park's edge that lead to private property. Either way, the two reconnect at the start of the Long Trail, marked in red, at roughly 0.5 mile overall.

From here the character of the trail begins to change. The trail is rockier and the forest more mature, and you feel as if you are hiking rather than strolling. In about 0.3 mile, intersect the Long Extension Trail on the left and the continuation of the Long Trail on the right.

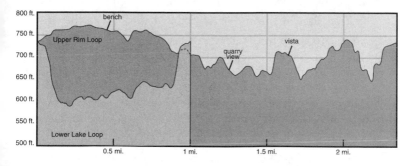

The Long Extension Trail heads farther northeast into the park and connects with the Powerline Trail, which skirts the eastern boundary of the park. Head south along the Long Trail and soon reach the intersection with the Pulpit Rock Loop, marked in yellow, on the left. Turn left and soon reach a small ledge along the trail that you will have to climb down. Around the eastern edge of the loop, you arrive at an intersection with a short crossover trail to the Powerline Trail, after which the trail swings west and intersects with the Saddle Back Trail, marked in red.

Take the Saddle Back Trail almost due south, a little less than 0.25 mile, and reach the blue-marked Lower Basin Trail. Bear left onto this trail and soon pass out of the forest into an opening created by the power lines that pass by the eastern edge of the park. Here a nice vista of a wetland lies to the east in an isolated portion of the park. The Powerline Trail heads northward here, while the Lower Basin Trail swings east.

Back along the loop, you soon come to the intersection with the crossover trail to the Lower Lake Loop, to the left. You could circumnavigate the lake at this point and avoid the steep stairs back to the parking area or skip the cliffside trail altogether, but I don't recommend it. The steep stairs are part of the experience, and the cliffside trail provides an interesting perspective on this deep plunge pool lake. Continue west, following blue paints, along what is now the Cliff Trail. Pass by the end of the Saddle Back Trail on the right and continue to climb to the intersection with the Long Trail. Here is where views of the lake down the steeply sided cliff really take on a dramatic perspective. Cedars and rock outcrops crowd the trail, providing a very different setting from the hardwood forest found elsewhere. But the setting is brief and the trail soon reaches the intersection with the Big Buck Trail, marked in white, and two options on how to descend along the Cliff Trail. Ahead is a short steep scramble, while to the right is a switchback. Both lead to the same point along the trail, so either choice is fine.

However you get there, the trail continues south, and you scramble to the top of another long portion of exposed rock beside the edge of the cliff. Glacier Lake lies more directly below you along this stretch of trail, and a chain-link fence shields hikers from the edge. Keep in mind that hikers, as elsewhere, are nearly directly below you on the lake trail. In no time you reach the parking area and the end of the 2.25-mile upper loop.

Lower Lake Loop

Before beginning a description of the Lower Lake Loop, it might be best to point out that the trail around the lake is rough. If not for the paints and its well-traversed path, I would categorize this part of the trail as a bushwhack. I mention this because most lakeside trails featured elsewhere in the book are relatively flat. Additionally, the stairs down to the lake are steep.

To reach the stairs to the Lower Lake Loop, head to the eastern edge of the parking lot, passing by the nature center on your right. Pass through another play area, and the steep stone stairs will be on the left. The stairs abruptly end practically on the lake's shore, and the route around the lake is a little hard to discern. For the most part, it is a narrow, worn path, but there are scrambles over logs and rocks (during the fall, leaves can often mask the trail). Likewise, the lake, depending on how high it is, can creep right up into the path. Otherwise you can find your way easily enough because the sheer cliff and lake are so close that there is virtually no other place to go than around. I recommend a clockwise direction, so you can take in the best scenery first, should you choose to return via the Cliff Trail instead of climbing the stairs.

Like Green and Round Lakes at Green Lakes State Park, described on page 58, Glacier Lake is a meromictic lake formed as a deep plunge pool at the base of a receding glacier. Looking up the steep cliff to your left, imagine the waterfall that carved through the cliff and 60 feet to the bottom of the lake.

The trail gets a little easier to follow along the northern edge and soon heads uphill and eastward as it navigates around the eastern marsh. At roughly the halfway point, 0.5 mile, you intersect the green-marked crossover trail that leads to the trails in the upper portion of the park. Shortly after, the trail crosses a stream and begins the return to the base of the stairs. The swamp accompanies you on the right for most of this return journey, with the lake coming into view just before you begin the steep ascent for a round-trip around the lake of 1 mile (3.25 miles if you included the Upper Rim Loop).

Nearby Attractions

Clark Reservation is of great interest to botanists due to the large number of unusual plants found within some special niches of the park. This is especially true for the estimated 19–23 different species of ferns. The park also features a native plant garden, with additional information about the park's remarkable plants available at the nature center, generally open mid-May–Labor Day.

Directions

From I-81, take Exit 16A for I-481 North. Merge onto I-481 North and get off on Exit 1 (Rock Cut Road), 0.5 mile. Turn right onto Rock Cut Road and follow it uphill to the light, 0.7 mile ahead. Turn left onto East Brighton Avenue, and continue straight through the light at 0.3 mile. East Brighton Avenue becomes NY 173 East/East Seneca Street, which you follow 1.8 miles south and then east. The entrance is on the left.

Baltimore Woods Nature Center

8

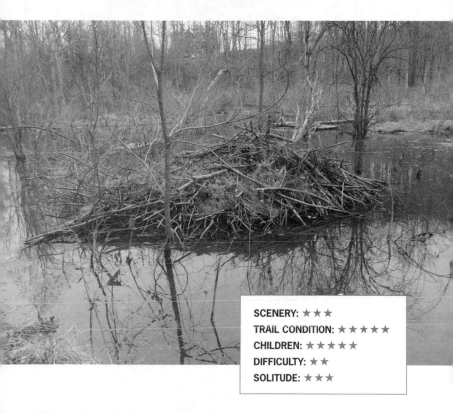

SCENERY: ★ ★ ★
TRAIL CONDITION: ★ ★ ★ ★ ★
CHILDREN: ★ ★ ★ ★ ★
DIFFICULTY: ★ ★
SOLITUDE: ★ ★ ★

GPS TRAILHEAD COORDINATES: N42° 57.919' W76° 20.642'

DISTANCE & CONFIGURATION: 2.5-mile loop; multiple side trails available

HIKING TIME: 1–2 hours

HIGHLIGHTS: Active beaver dam, woodland stroll

ELEVATION: 830' at trailhead, 720' at lowest point along trail

ACCESS: Daily, sunrise–sunset; no fees or permits required

MAPS: baltimorewoods.org/visit/interpretive-center-trails; also available at information kiosks on-site

FACILITIES: Visitor center, picnic area, restrooms in visitor center when open

WHEELCHAIR ACCESS: No

COMMENTS: No dogs allowed

CONTACTS: Baltimore Woods Nature Center, 315-673-1350, **baltimorewoods.org**

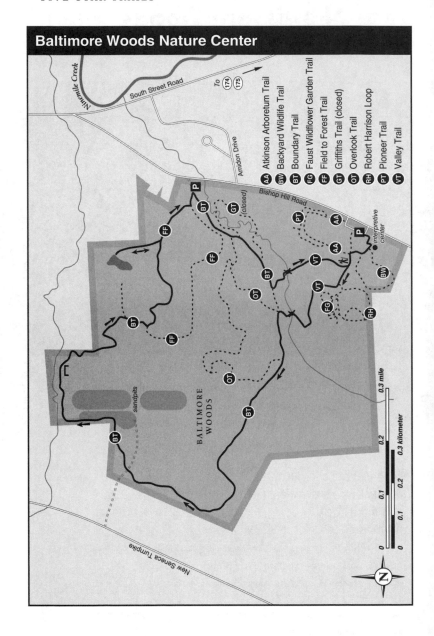

Baltimore Woods Nature Center

AA Atkinson Arboretum Trail
BW Backyard Wildlife Trail
BT Boundary Trail
FG Faust Wildflower Garden Trail
FF Field to Forest Trail
GT Griffiths Trail (closed)
OT Overlook Trail
RH Robert Harrison Loop
PT Pioneer Trail
VT Valley Trail

Overview

For such a small park, Baltimore Woods packs a lot of great hiking features in its 182 acres. Varied terrain, distinct habitats, and lots of wildlife activity make it an excellent trip. The beaver activity near the lower parking area is especially interesting. Evidence of their dam building is present along a portion of the Boundary Trail and has even led to closure of the Griffiths Trail since significant portions of the trail have become submerged.

Route Details

The trail described includes sections along multiple routes and is sequenced as follows: Valley Trail (yellow), Boundary Trail (pink), Field to Forest Trail (Green), Boundary Trail (Pink), and Valley Trail (yellow). The trails are superbly maintained and marked, so finding your way is easy even if you choose to explore a different route than detailed here. There are also several shorter options for families with very young children. These flat, shorter nature trails are near the nature center and include the Backyard Wildlife Trail (blue, 0.3 mile), Atkinson Arboretum Trail (green, 0.4 mile), Faust Wildflower Garden Trail (purple, mileage varies), Robert Harrison Loop (tan, 0.15 mile), and Pioneer Trail (red, 0.3 mile). None of these shorter trails is included in the route here, which would certainly be a good choice

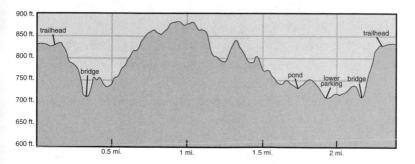

for children as well, despite a couple of steep sections. Many benches are situated along the trails and provide excellent opportunities for visitors to simply enjoy the setting.

To reach the trailhead from the upper parking area, head straight across the open lawn toward the stand of pine trees in the southeast corner, past the pavilion. Look for the Valley Trail, marked with yellow diamonds. This is the start and end of the loop, and you will want to continue straight, the left choice and westward. Very quickly the overall feel of the trail transitions from a park setting into a deep woodland. Surrounded by a mature hardwood forest, the trail descends, weaving its way along the contours of the hill approximately 0.25 mile down to a small stream crossed by a wooden bridge. On the other side of the bridge you reach a major trail intersection. To your right is the continuation of the Valley Trail and Boundary Trail. Straight ahead is a portion of the orange Overlook Trail, while to your left is the rest of the Overlook Trail and the path we are headed down, the pink Boundary Trail.

Turn left and follow the Boundary Trail, briefly marked with both orange and pink placards. Soon after this turn, cross a culvert, after which the orange trail diverts to the right, while the Boundary Trail continues straight ahead. There are no more intersections for a while, and you can focus on the trail and not the map. The trail begins to climb 100 feet over the next 0.5 mile, and though the ascent is not steep, it is steady. You soon pass a small plantation of pines on your left, and the trail opens into rolling fields and abandoned orchards. You are approximately 0.75 mile from the parking area, which is slightly hard to believe as the changes in terrain and habitat make it feel more spread out.

Around the 1-mile marker, you intersect an access road coming in from the left. This road leads to an old borrow pit, which is an excavation of sand, gravel, or soil that is used elsewhere for construction. This particular borrow pit is a sandpit that once provided supplementary income to farmers. Much of the landscape in Central New York and Baltimore Woods is riddled with these pits as glacial deposits often left sorted layers of sand or gravel. Deposits of glacial till beside glaciers and adjoining valleys formed mounds called kames. Related to kames are kettles, which were also formed by glacial deposits. Unlike kames, kettles contained significant quantities of ice. When the ice melted thousands of years ago, it left depressions that later filled to create shallow lakes. A combination of kames and kettles forms the hummocky topography and rolling hills found at Baltimore Woods.

Head straight across this intersection and up a short hill above the sandpit along a meandering and narrow footpath. The trail continues out in the open for another 0.3 mile before reentering the woods, just after passing a cornfield. The active cornfield is part of the park's management plan to maintain portions of open field rather than letting the landscape become entirely woodland. Where you reenter the forest, you are approximately halfway along the loop. Descend toward the stream, where a pair of benches faces the stream and furnishes an excellent stopping point to linger. Past the benches, the trail turns southward and briefly uphill over a small knoll before weaving its way eastward through the forest. The trail descends through a switchback and soon after intersects with the Field to Forest Trail, marked with green diamonds. Continue left, now following the green diamonds, and you soon come into sight of a small pond off to your left, just before the trail enters an open field. A side trail to the pond just a short way ahead is another pleasant diversion. It is less than 0.1 mile to visit the pond.

Continuing along the mowed green trail, you soon reach an intersection with a trail on your right. Continue past this a short way to the lower parking area. As you return along the Boundary Trail, the evidence of the beavers' prolific activity can be seen throughout. Dams, chewed stumps, and downed trees are striking evidence of nature's busy builders and hydrological engineers. The beaver came to the park in 2005, and as its activity continues, you cannot help but wonder how much more rerouting of the trail network here will be necessary.

To return to the upper parking area, continue southwest along the Boundary Trail, though markings are sporadic. The beaver activity here is the most widespread, and you will see several trail markers remaining out in the backwater where a trail once existed. Our route passes an intersection with the green trail on your right, shortly followed by an old gravel pit and the old intersection with Griffiths Trail in short succession. The Griffiths Trail has become submerged in the backwaters of recent beaver activity and is essentially closed. At 2.2 miles, you re-intersect the yellow-marked Valley Trail that leads back to the upper parking area. Bear left and downhill, and then cross a wooden bridge over the stream. When I visited the trail, beavers had recently been active in this area. Shortly after crossing the stream, the trail climbs 100 feet over the next 0.25 mile and is the steepest section of trail. The good news is that, on reaching the top, you are practically back at your car for a round-trip of 2.5 miles.

Directions

From points east of Marcellus: Heading west along NY 175 West/West Seneca Turnpike, continue straight onto NY 174/East Main Street. Turn left onto South State Street; go 0.5 mile. Turn right onto CR 211/Bishop Hill Road; travel 0.5 mile. The upper parking area is 0.6 mile ahead on your right.

From points west of Marcellus: Follow US 20/East Genesee Street east and bear left onto NY 175 East/Lee-Mulroy Road. At 2.3 miles, turn left onto CR 211/Bishop Hill Road. The upper parking area is 1 mile ahead on your left.

9 Rattlesnake Gulf & Adams Eden Camp

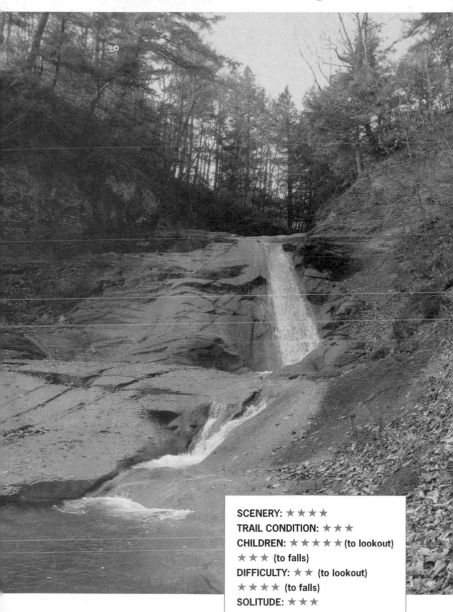

SCENERY: ★ ★ ★ ★
TRAIL CONDITION: ★ ★ ★
CHILDREN: ★ ★ ★ ★ ★ (to lookout)
★ ★ ★ (to falls)
DIFFICULTY: ★ ★ (to lookout)
★ ★ ★ ★ (to falls)
SOLITUDE: ★ ★ ★

Rattlesnake Gulf & Adams Eden Camp

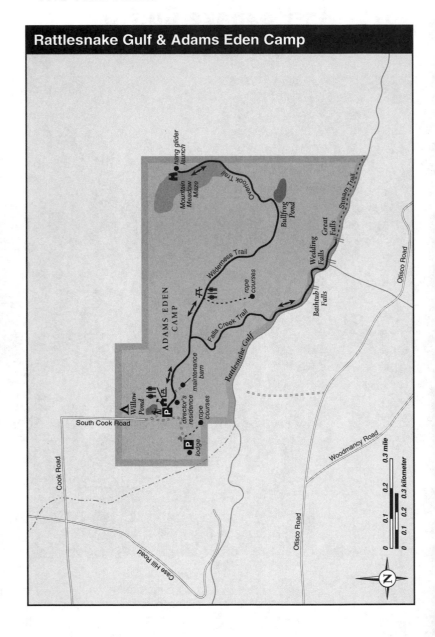

GPS TRAILHEAD COORDINATES: N42° 52.165' W76° 10.611'

DISTANCE & CONFIGURATION: 2.5-mile out-and-back to hang glider launch; 1.6-mile out-and-back side trip to base of Great Falls

HIKING TIME: 1–2 hours

HIGHLIGHTS: Panoramic view, waterfalls

ELEVATION: 1,250' at trailhead; 1,469' at hang glider launch; 786' at base of Great Falls

ACCESS: Wednesday–Monday, 9 a.m.–sunset; $4 individual, $8 family. Falls Creek Trail is open late spring–late fall but is closed during times of heavy runoff, so call ahead if you wish to visit that trail.

MAPS: adamsedencamp.com/about-us/camp-map; also available on-site

FACILITIES: Ropes course, GPS course, picnic area, campgrounds, restrooms

WHEELCHAIR ACCESS: No

COMMENTS: The trail system at Adams Eden is on private property. All visitors must register upon entering the property, and there are special rules and regulations about activities permitted. A full list of rules and regulations is available upon registration or online at **adamsedencamp.com/about-us/camp-policies.** Dogs allowed on leash only.

CONTACTS: Adams Eden Camp, 315-677-5121, **adamsedencamp.com**

Overview

Unique to the hikes featured in this book, Rattlesnake Gulf and the trail to the hang glider launch are on private property. As such, permitted activities are slightly more restrictive than those at public parks (see **adamsedencamp.com/about-us/camp-policies** for rules). But also distinctive from most other trails in the region are the stunning

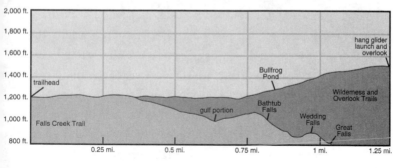

panoramic views at the hang glider launch and the bushwhack-like creek walk within the gorge.

Route Details

Overlook Trail

The path to the Overlook Trail follows the camp's maintenance roads, and though the route itself is pretty unremarkable, the view at the top is anything but. From the parking area and registration office, head southeast along the main road past the maintenance buildings. This is the designated beginning of the trail system, but really it is just a continuation of the camp access roads. Start along the Wilderness Trail, and in less than 0.3 mile pass the Falls Creek Trail, via the Middle Meadow Trail, on your right. For now continue straight along the main road, Wilderness Trail, passing one of two ropes courses found on the property on the right. At a little over 0.75 mile, reach Bullfrog Pond and the intersection with Overlook Trail. Though the hike has had some rolling terrain, from here the climbing begins in earnest. The Overlook Trail climbs 200 feet over the next 0.4 mile. Painted wood trail markers with a rising sun, as well as other posters, lead the way. Pass the Mountain Meadow Maze on your left, and soon after, at 1.25 miles, reach the hang glider launch and overlook after passing through an open field.

Here you will find the one thing lacking along most of the trails found in the region: a truly panoramic view. Despite reaching the lookout on an overcast and hazy day, I could see for miles to the east and north. Once again the transformative powers of the last glacial period of the ice age are evident. As found throughout the region, steep sloped hills of nearly identical height sprawl out as far as the eye can see. In between are broad, nearly flat U-shaped valleys, but no rivers or streams are present. Instead, the bulldozing power of great ice sheets scoured the hills, flattened the troughs, and wiped away earlier signs of the typical V-shaped valleys formed by erosion. Return the way you came for a round-trip of 2.5 miles, or add the creek walk described below to include some real adventure to your trip.

Falls Creek Trail (Rattlesnake Gulf)

Before beginning the stream trail, a few words of caution are in order. The trail is a creek walk and has many steep and difficult sections to traverse. The property owners strongly emphasize that you be in "good physical condition" to attempt the creek walk. I wholeheartedly agree. Expect to get wet and/or muddy, and do not attempt this hike unless you have proper footwear and are confident in your ability to walk along wet and slippery surfaces. Be aware that within the creek bed, conditions often change, and sections that were once solid can be undercut or become heavily eroded. Move slowly, check your footing, and do not attempt during rainy or flood conditions. It is also recommended that you do not attempt this trip solo. Furthermore, the camp owns only a portion of the property along the creek, so be mindful of posted signs and do not trespass.

From the Wilderness Trail, follow the Middle Meadow Trail through the open field by bearing to your left, and soon pass through a section of the second ropes course. From here on, the trail begins a much steeper descent, roughly 250 feet over the next 0.25 mile. Steps, rope railings, and some steep scrambles have to be navigated before reaching the streambed below. Note that the trail leading upstream is closed, and following it will result in immediate expulsion from the property. Across the stream is a sign noting that a nearby firing range uses live rounds, so it's best to turn left and stay on the north side of the creek.

Pick your way along streambed boulders and gravelly shores for about 0.3 mile to the first of the two major falls along the creek walk. You may have noted Bathtub Falls, a flume with a rectangular pool below, a little ways back, but Wedding Falls is the first cascade that would be qualified as a waterfall. Over a dozen feet high, the cascade surges along the left side, so you'll have to navigate your way down

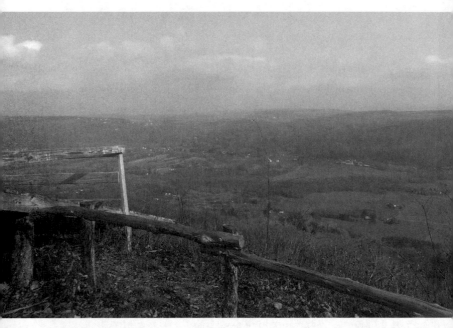

HANG GLIDER LAUNCH

the right-hand side of the stream. (*Note:* Left and right are given facing downstream.)

A short distance farther southeast, the stream and trail reach the abrupt edge of Great Falls, a bifurcated falls roughly 25 feet tall. It is a steep drop-off, and at this point you'll have to assess conditions and your nerve to continue on. To reach the base of the falls, look to the left, where a set of steps are cut into the crumbly shale that leads to a narrow ledge and eventually a scramble down the steep hillside. Ropes are set into the shale to assist you, but because the shale is crumbly, test the rope before putting weight against it. Though the route is navigable, I would not recommend it for anyone who has doubts.

Beyond the base of the falls, the trail continues downstream. However, the creek walk farther downstream is very difficult and potentially dangerous. Many sections are actively eroding, with one section covered by a rockslide and another by a mud/clay slide. At the clay slide, the stream is almost completely dammed, and the entire route is along slippery and eroding clay deposits. The scene here is catastrophic. Boulders, tree trunks, and huge slides of clay intermix, making a very treacherous spot. If you do attempt to continue, expect a pound or two of clay to stick to your boots. After crossing these difficult sections, the stream reverts back to a deeply incised gorge, and though scenic, it's not worth the effort or risk. A couple tiny falls and flumes are found down this section, but certainly Great Falls is the gem along this trip. I would not recommend the trip farther down to even the most diehard hikers. Rather, spend some time enjoying Great Falls and return the way you came for a round-trip of 1.6 miles, 4.1 miles if you also included the Overlook Trail.

Nearby Attractions

Adams Eden Camp is in the heart of Syracuse's outlying apple orchards. During the fall, apple picking is one of many activities available at the stalls, stores, and orchards that dot US 20. Also showcased are fresh-baked goods, crafts, locally grown food, and hayrides and other outdoor activities. Though the trail will be fun anytime, you might want to plan your trip to coincide with the fall picking season to take advantage of all that the orchard valleys have to offer.

Directions

From I-81 take Exit 15, Lafayette/US 20 West. Take US 20 West/Cherry Valley Turnpike 4.3 miles west, and turn left on Case Hill Road. Follow it 2.3 miles and turn left onto Cook Road. Continue 0.6 mile to the Adams Eden Camp entrance on the left.

10 Highland Forest: Phil Suters Memorial Main Trail

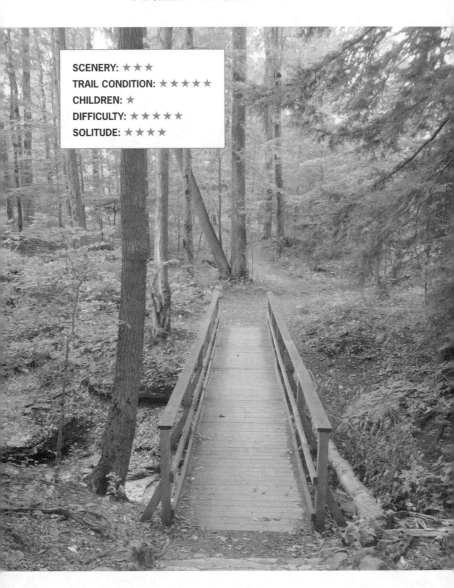

SCENERY: ★ ★ ★
TRAIL CONDITION: ★ ★ ★ ★ ★
CHILDREN: ★
DIFFICULTY: ★ ★ ★ ★ ★
SOLITUDE: ★ ★ ★ ★

GPS TRAILHEAD COORDINATES: N42° 50.199'   W75° 55.394'

DISTANCE & CONFIGURATION: 8.8-mile loop

HIKING TIME: 4–5 hours

HIGHLIGHTS: Secluded woodland

ELEVATION: 1,665' at trailhead; 1,941' at highest point along loop; multiple changes in elevation

ACCESS: March–November: Daily, 8:30 a.m.–5:30 p.m. December–February: Daily, 8:30 a.m.–4:30 p.m.; $3 per person

MAPS: onondagacountyparks.com/highland-forest

FACILITIES: Restrooms, water sources, visitor center, trail shelters

WHEELCHAIR ACCESS: No

COMMENTS: Portions of the trail are shared with equestrians and mountain bikers.

CONTACTS: Highland Forest Park, 315-683-5550, **onondagacountyparks.com /highland-forest**

Overview

Long loop trails are hard to find in the region, but the Phil Suters Memorial Main Trail around Highland Forest is among those treasured few. Though a popular destination, this trail proves that distance is the best assurance for solitude. You will definitely encounter people along the trails but only in passing. The trail system here is a veritable maze of intersecting hiking/skiing and biking trails. There are shorter options available and, more important, many alternative routes to explore on your own for future visits.

Route Details

The Phil Suters Memorial Main Trail circumnavigates the 2,729-acre park. All along this trek are intersections with access roads, skid trails, horse trails, and biking/skiing trails, as well as shorter hiking loops. Indeed, along some sections it seems that there is nothing but intersections. In short, the park is a veritable maze, albeit a very well-marked one. When describing other trails, intersections are often a good reference to gauge progress, yet this trail has so many that intersections are more confusing than helpful. Furthermore, the network

Highland Forest: Phil Suters Memorial Main Trail

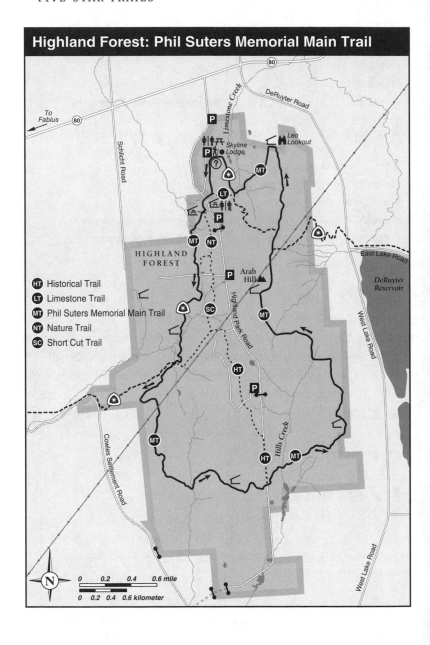

Legend:
- **HT** Historical Trail
- **LT** Limestone Trail
- **MT** Phil Suters Memorial Main Trail
- **NT** Nature Trail
- **SC** Short Cut Trail

of hiking/snowshoe trails is not the same as those for biking/skiing. The biking/skiing trails are outlined on a different map than the hiking map and often share small portions of the same route. Both maps are available in the Skyline Lodge. Though they may share similar colors, note that hiking/snowshoe trails are designated with squares, while biking/skiing trails use diamonds. Rather than providing droll descriptions of each intersection, I will try to keep the information to the bare minimum required to keep you on track and along the desired path. More often than not, you simply head straight across most intersections, which for the most part are clearly indicated. Thus I have highlighted only those intersections of significance to the hiker and omitted many for other outdoor recreationists. Also, the park has many reference points (for example, 27A) indicated on the map and found along the trail. Mileage back to the main parking area is often noted at the trail intersection, so you can best gauge your progress. Rest assured the network is more problematic in description than in navigation.

From the parking area beside Skyline Lodge, head to the information kiosk, clearly labeled "Trails," at the southern edge of the lot. To the left of the kiosk, identified by a large green-and-white lettered sign, is the beginning of the Phil Suters Memorial Main Trail. The trail is well marked with orange square placards and begins along

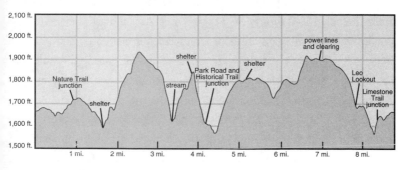

a level and broad cut through a pine plantation. Continue across the main park road and pass by a picnic shelter. After about 0.3 mile you pass an interesting signboard, where, in addition to park maps, is a clock and temperature gauge. An additional sign states that, from this point, the main loop is 8.7 miles long. Pass this sign and cross over a wood bridge, where you'll finally begin to feel as if you are on a hiking trail rather than strolling within a park. The western leg of the Main Trail shares sections with the Nature (1.86-mile loop), Short Cut (3.6-mile loop), and Historical (7.76-mile loop) hiking trails. As the sign indicates, their departure from the Main Trail is shown, not the sections that they share. In those circumstances all are marked with the orange squares of the Main Trail. In addition to the orange squares, you may also notice some blue paints. These are not indications of a separate trail within the park, but in fact are part of the North Country Trail (NCT) that weaves its way from North Dakota to New York. (For more information, see **nctacnychapter.org**.)

At 0.9 mile the Nature Trail, marked in green, departs to the left and heads back north toward the main parking area. A short way ahead, you reach the first bike/ski trail that bisects the hiking trail (note the diamond versus square placard). Past this intersection you traverse a built-up section of the trail, where a gravel base is enclosed in landscape timbers. As you head downhill the atmosphere begins to take on a progressively more wilderness feel. The trail descends approximately 150 feet over the next 0.5 mile. As you reach the end of the descent, you will pass an extra-long picnic table situated before a trail shelter on your right. This shelter, like the others along the trail, has a map inside and is for day-use only; camping within the park is prohibited. You are not yet a quarter of the way along the circuit, and though this appears an excellent spot to stop, it may be a little early. There is another shelter ahead, about a mile short of the halfway point, as well as another shelter around the 5-mile point. Although these latter shelters are more convenient stopping points, this one has the most pleasant setting.

Cross the wooden bridge over the stream in front of the shelter, and begin climbing roughly 350 feet over just shy of a mile. Soon after beginning the climb, the Short Cut Trail, designated by black and yellow placards, diverts to the left; stay to your right, continuing to follow the orange squares. After a series of switches, bridges, descents, and stream crossings, the trail takes a sharp left turn beside a sign labeled "Easy Street."

To the right/straight the North Country Trail heads off east, while the Main Trail continues uphill and to the south. The gradual climb follows a broad grassy road with a worn path through its center; continue another 300 feet over the next 0.6 mile to complete the ascent that you began at the first trail shelter. The summit, 1,941 feet and the highest point along the trail, is essentially marked by the swath cut by the power line that passes through the forest here. The path continues along the hilltop a brief way and soon reaches a fork in the trail. To the left is the continuation of the Main Trail, while to your right is an unmarked grassy road. Past this fork, the trail begins a 300-foot descent over the next mile.

Shortly after completing a switchback, you reach a stream crossing and the end of the descent. Rock-hop across the stream and begin to climb much of the elevation just descended, 200 feet of gain over the next 0.5 mile. At the time I hiked the trail, the forest had been recently thinned, and skid trails intersected and joined sections of the Main Trail along this ascent. Disturbances caused by logging and skid trails usually revert back to a natural state within a couple of years, but the path here will likely appear quite broad for years to come.

The winding ascent ends at around 3.8 miles at a major intersection along the loop and in front of the second trail shelter. Bisecting the trail in the north-south direction is the light purple South Extension bike/ski trail. Continue heading east; after crossing an intersection with a horse trail, the trail begins another descent. The trail descends a little less than 300 feet over the next 0.5 mile. The decline is steep at first but begins to slacken a bit as you pass through abandoned orchards. Just over 4 miles overall, you reach an intersection with the Main Park Road and the departure of the Historical Trail, identified by brown squares. Both road and trail head northward back to the park office. For most of the remaining trail, which continues straight ahead, you will pass many intersections, but almost none of them will be with hiking trails but rather roads, horse trails, and bike/ski trails.

Across the road, the Main Trail continues to descend as it passes through a section of mostly pines where a thick understory crowds the trail. As you reach the bottom of this descent, the trail enters a wet area where corduroy and short bridges weave through a floodplain along Hills Creek. Old apple trees are interspersed along the creek, making an excellent attraction for wildlife. Once across the creek, the trail begins to climb once again. Though it's not the last climb along the trail, it is the last protracted one, with over 225 feet of elevation gain in the next 0.5 mile.

The trail eventually levels off after passing a horse-trail intersection and soon reaches the third trail shelter among a dense stand of pines, at roughly 5 miles. A major intersection of several biking trails is here. Coming in from your left and continuing on your right is the Southside Loop marked with orange diamonds, not to be confused with the Main Trail, marked with orange squares, that also heads northward and slightly to your right but essentially straight ahead.

Continue straight ahead, through a dense stand of spruce, and pass through some wet areas along the trail. The trail briefly re-intersects the Southside Loop before diverging off to your left just past reference marker 16C. You soon intersect a road and join it heading westward as you dip down to a small stream crossing. Across the stream you climb first northerly before the trail swings westward along a broad road, where you again intersect the Southside Loop. The two continue westward together a brief way before diverging from each other in a small clearing in the forest.

Continue to your right, and begin a climb that nearly summits Arab Hill. This begins the final northward trek back to the parking area. Along this passage there are many intersections with horse trails, roads, and various ski/bike trails. You pass through a clearing in the forest, where power lines again cut a broad swath through the forest, 6.6 miles total along the trail. Just past this opening the trail rejoins the North Country Trail for a brief while. At 7.2 miles, begin a 300-foot descent over the next 0.75 mile. The descent begins steeply and then levels off briefly where it intersects a bike trail and passes by the final trail shelter near Leo Lookout. The lookout abuts the park's northern boundary, and the view is partially obstructed by some trees downhill on private property. Past the shelter the trail takes a sharp left and continues to descend the last 120 feet to where the trail crosses Limestone Creek. The trail begins the final ascent heading westward but turns sharply right when you intersect the Limestone Trail, marked in pink. The remaining trek northward passes quickly, and you soon reach the outlying lawns beside Skyline Lodge, for a total trip length of 8.8 miles.

Directions

From I-81, take Exit 14 (NY 80/NY 11A/Tully). Turn onto NY 80 East, and follow it east 11 miles to CR 188/Highland Park Road. Turn right and travel 1 mile. Turn right and follow the signs to Skyline Lodge.

11 # Tinker Falls & Jones Hill

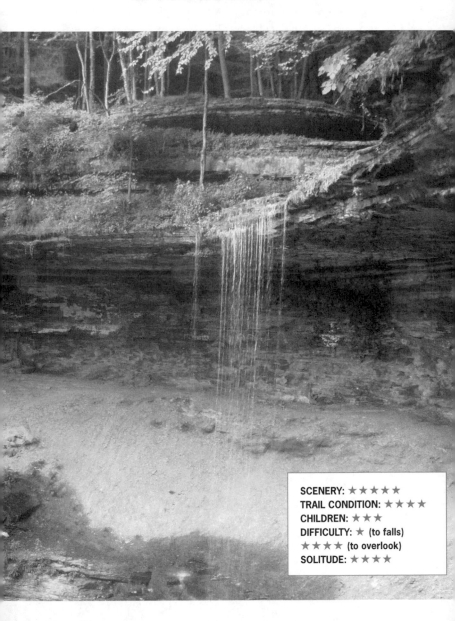

SCENERY: ★ ★ ★ ★ ★
TRAIL CONDITION: ★ ★ ★ ★
CHILDREN: ★ ★ ★
DIFFICULTY: ★ (to falls)
★ ★ ★ ★ (to overlook)
SOLITUDE: ★ ★ ★ ★

GPS TRAILHEAD COORDINATES: N42° 46.801'   W76° 02.144'

DISTANCE & CONFIGURATION: 0.5-mile out-and-back to Tinker Falls; 2.0-mile out-and-back to hang glider lookout; 2.5-mile total for both

HIKING TIME: 1–2 hours

HIGHLIGHTS: Waterfall, hang glider launch, scenic vista

ELEVATION: 1,250' at trailhead; 1,900' at scenic overlook; no significant rise to Tinker Falls

ACCESS: Open 24/7; no fees or permits required

MAPS: DEC Labrador Hollow Unique Area map: **dec.ny.gov/lands/37349.html**; Finger Lakes Trail Conference: Sheet O1

FACILITIES: None

WHEELCHAIR ACCESS: Yes to Tinker Falls; no to scenic overlook

COMMENTS: The trip to view Tinker Falls is accessible, but the trip to the hang glider launch and scenic overlook is not. Unlike at other Department of Environmental Conservation lands, camping and fires are prohibited in the Labrador Hollow Unique Area.

CONTACTS: NYSDEC Region 7, Cortland Sub-Office, 607-753-3095, **dec.ny.gov/lands/37070.html**

Overview

The trip to Tinker Falls is a short, flat stroll beside Tinker Falls Creek. Be especially careful exploring the area around the falls, as the crumbling shale is steep and slippery. Add some difficulty and a scenic vista to your trip by heading to the nearby hang glider launchpad. Though the climb to the launchpad is steep at times, it is certainly worth the effort.

Route Details

Tinker Falls Trail

There are two parking areas near the trailhead. One small area is on the east side of NY 91 for those with accessibility needs, but most hikers should plan to use the much larger parking area on the western side of the road. The trail to Tinker Falls is just past the Labrador Hollow Unique Area information kiosk, located on the north side of the accessible parking area. The path is broad and wheelchair accessible and features a couple of benches along the 0.25-mile stroll to the falls. In no time you'll see the looming falls ahead, though depending on

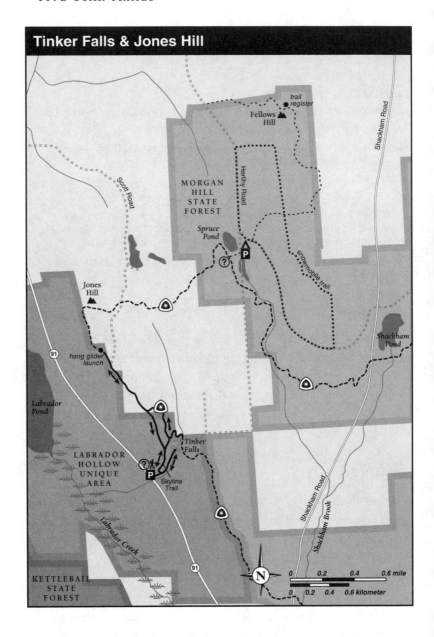

Tinker Falls & Jones Hill

the time of year, you may not hear the telltale sounds of a waterfall. Tinker Falls Creek is seasonal, so to see the 50-foot "hanging" waterfall in all its glory, plan your visit after a recent rain and especially during the spring melt. The accessible trail ends far below and a few hundred feet south of the waterfall. But, as is evident by the numerous paths on the opposing bank, other explorers regularly continue onward and climb the crumbly shale slopes and proceed up to the deep cavernous overhang that lies behind the falls. At 100 feet wide, 30 feet deep, and 30 feet high, it is a popular spot and unfortunately one that is often covered with graffiti, a rather pointless gesture since the shale readily erodes and washes away the offending marks. The deep shelf illustrates the stark contrast between the erosion-resistant Tully capstone and the relatively fragile shale beneath, essential for the falls' atypical formation.

Jones Hill Trail

To view the falls from above and reach the hang glider lookout, return the way you came. About halfway back, you will see a fork in the trail with a path leading westward and uphill on your right. Head up this short hill to an intersection with the hang glider access road. The road, the Skyline Trail, is marked with pale orange paint and heads uphill, to your right, at an ever steepening grade. Roughly 0.1 mile along the climb, you reach a fork in the road and a bit of confusion about the

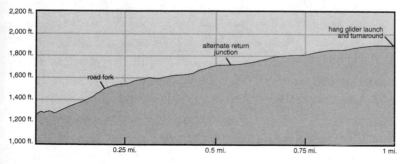

direction of the trail. The hang glider access road continues uphill to the left, while the orange blazes continue uphill on the right. However, as you reach the point where the trail levels off, a Department of Environmental Conservation yellow warning sign, reading "No Trespassing for Any Reason," directly faces you. Based on the angle of the sign, it seems to indicate that the trail ahead (or at least this section) is closed. Yet this sign is meant to make you avoid the steep and fragile slope of the gorge on the right and not keep you from continuing along the trail, straight ahead. The orientation of this sign is unfortunate, as it likely makes many hikers turn back and follow the hang glider access road to the scenic overlook rather than the designated forest trail. Both will get you there and both are on state land, but the broad road—which we join later on—is not particularly interesting and, in my opinion, takes away from the experience. Furthermore, you will miss the opportunity to view the falls from above and take in a truly spectacular view. Note that if you choose the road over the trail, the distance is marginally less but much steeper.

To follow the trail, continue past the yellow warning sign and follow the orange blazes a short distance to where the Skyline Trail ends and intersects the Onondaga/North Country Trail. The blue Onondaga Trail is a spur trail for the white Finger Lakes Trail and both are sections along the North Country Trail (NCT), a 4,600-mile trek from North Dakota to New York.

For now, follow the trail, marked in blue, straight ahead another 0.25 mile and take a series of switchbacks to reach the top of Tinker Falls. The view down to the washed-out amphitheater is actually a bit dizzying, so I don't recommend it for anyone with a fear of heights or a touch of vertigo. Extreme caution should be used if you choose to view the falls from above. As you observed from below, there are no slopes around these falls, only a vertical drop from the hanging ledge.

This side trail continues past the top of Tinker Falls and into the southern portion of Morgan Hill State Forest. A combination of the Onondaga Trail/NCT and roads within the state forest could provide extended and even overnight trips for those who wish for additional challenges. See the Morgan Hill State Forest: Fellows Hill Loop featured on page 105 for one of these longer trips.

Return to where the Skyline Trail intersects the Onondaga Trail/NCT, turn right to go northward, and follow the Onondaga Trail, marked with blue paint blazes, to reach the overlook. The trail is now the standard footpath with which many hikers are familiar and is very similar to hiking trails in the Adirondacks. Indeed the Labrador Hollow Unique Area is notable for its similarities to the Adirondacks, especially around Labrador Pond (see description in Nearby Attractions). The trail steadily climbs among beech and maple trees, with an especially steep climb and switchback about 0.25 mile along this segment.

Shortly after the switchback, you will pass an odd maple tree that forks near its base to form an empty cavity just above the soil. This odd tree stands beside the trail and is within a few short strides of the re-intersection with the steep access road.

The designated trail turns right to follow the access road a short way, and then turns back into the forest along a blue-marked trail. You can follow the access road all the way to the overlook, but as mentioned earlier the trails provide a little more variety.

The next leg of the trail is probably the only place you might encounter a few muddy areas, so bypassing this section of trail while following the road might be advisable during wet and rainy conditions. The footpath briefly winds its way westward before re-intersecting and then crossing the access road. Head straight across the road, south, and continue to follow the blue paint blazes. If you have chosen to follow the road for portions or most of the hike, now is the optimal time to rejoin the trail. In autumn when the foliage is less dense, you will have less obstructed views of the valley below. At 1 mile from the trailhead, it is as if you suddenly pop out of the surrounding forest into a small clearing along the hilltop. This open lawn is often referred to as Jones Hill, though the actual hilltop is farther northwest along the Fellows Hill Loop. Spreading out before you is the narrow valley, 0.5-mile wide, that encompasses the Labrador

Hollow Unique Area, whose pond, parking area, and main information center lie some 700 feet below. This spectacular view and the small clearing allow for a unique perspective on the rolling, forested hills of the Finger Lakes and Central New York region. If you want to extend your excursion, continue on to the Fellows Hill Loop hike described on the following pages.

Nearby Attractions

North of the trailhead parking area is Labrador Pond, a boat launch, and a wetland boardwalk. This special area provides additional wheelchair-accessible areas as well as fishing and boating opportunities. Labrador Hollow is nestled between two steep hillsides that effectively shade the area most of the day. Consequently the microclimate in this valley is more similar to Adirondack bogs than to the open valleys typical in the region. If you visit the area and some of your party doesn't want to make the trip up to the hang glider launchpad, they could spend a pleasant afternoon here and also have the chance to glimpse the rest of the hiking group at the scenic overlook high above.

Directions

From the north: From the intersection of NY 80 and NY 91, just east of Apulia Station, turn onto NY 91 South/Apulia-Truxton Road. Head south 3.3 miles, past Labrador Cross Road and the Labrador Hollow Unique Area complex, to the large pulloff on the west side of the road.

From the south: From the intersection of NY 13 and NY 91 in Truxton, turn onto NY 91 North/Apulia-Truxton Road. Head north 5 miles to the large pulloff on the west side of the road.

12 # Morgan Hill State Forest: Fellows Hill Loop

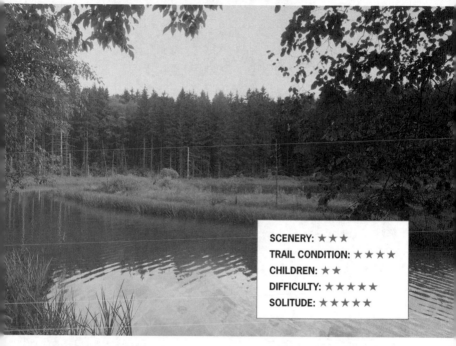

SCENERY: ★ ★ ★
TRAIL CONDITION: ★ ★ ★ ★
CHILDREN: ★ ★
DIFFICULTY: ★ ★ ★ ★ ★
SOLITUDE: ★ ★ ★ ★ ★

GPS TRAILHEAD COORDINATES: (Tinker Falls trailhead) N42° 46.801' W76° 02.144'

DISTANCE & CONFIGURATION: 6.0-mile balloon from the end of the Tinker Falls & Jones Hill trail; 8.0-mile balloon overall

HIKING TIME: 2.5–3.5 hours

HIGHLIGHTS: Isolated woodland, pond

ELEVATION: 1,250' at Tinker Falls trailhead; 1,900' at hang glider launch; 2,000' at Fellows Hill

ACCESS: Open 24/7; no fees or permits required

MAPS: DEC Morgan Hill State Forest map: **dec.ny.gov/lands/37346.html**; Finger Lakes Trail Conference: Sheet 01

FACILITIES: None

WHEELCHAIR ACCESS: No

COMMENTS: This trail begins and ends with the Tinker Falls & Jones Hill trail described on page 98.

CONTACTS: NYSDEC Region 7, Cortland Sub-Office, 607-753-3095, **dec.ny.gov /lands/37115.html**

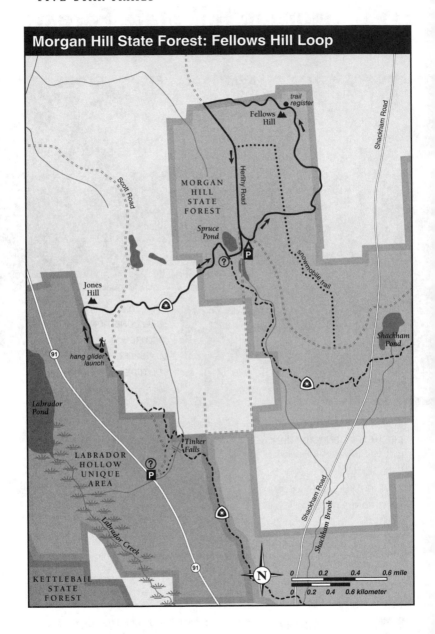

Morgan Hill State Forest: Fellows Hill Loop

Overview

The steep climb to Jones Hill will provide a nice warm-up for the longer and more difficult Fellows Hill Loop. Unfortunately Fellows Hill does not have the stunning view that the hang glider launch near Jones Hill does, but the variety of terrain and ecosystems found along this extended trip will prove rewarding nonetheless.

Route Details

Once you've finished taking in the sights at the hang glider launch (see Tinker Falls & Jones Hill Trail, page 98), look to the north for an opening in a dense thicket of beech trees that encircles the clearing. The path, marked with blue paints, is near the steep drop-off and appears narrow but widens within the forest. (*Note:* Trail mileage will be given from the hang glider launch forward, but overall progress will include an additional mile.) The trail continues northward about 0.25 mile along the steep hillside before turning east. At this point the trail departs from state land and enters onto private property for the next 0.9 mile. As usual, respect the property owners' generous offer of granting access by remaining on the trail. The trail experiences a slight but steady decline and soon crosses an overgrown access road, after which the decline steepens and follows switchbacks down to a crossing over Tinker Falls Creek. A forest road intersects the stream crossing as

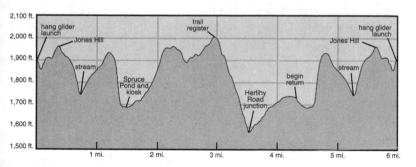

well, but the trail is clearly marked in blue directly across the stream. Once you've rock-hopped across the stream and made your way over the opposing bank, you cross another forest road and make a second stream crossing. After the second crossing, you begin a 160-foot climb over the next 0.5 mile. You begin to pass through a spruce forest as you near the top of your ascent, but no sooner than you reach the apex, the trail begins a much steeper descent to Spruce Pond. Though very steep in some sections (a 250-foot elevation loss in less than 0.25 mile), the trail is in good condition with switchbacks to ease the descent. Indeed, with all the ascents and descents along this loop, it would make an excellent conditioning trail when compared to the mostly level trails typical in the region.

At the bottom, the trail reaches Spruce Pond and turns sharply southward. The trail follows the western shore of the pond within feet of the water; near the pond's southern end you reach a fork in the trail and a small kiosk with information about the North Country Trail (NCT). The NCT/Onondaga Trail continues straight ahead, marked in blue, while the Fellows Hill Loop and Spruce Pond parking area are on the left. Turn left and head east over the berm that forms the southern edge of Spruce Pond. At the berm's conclusion, the trail passes through a gravel parking area beside Herlihy Road. Bear left and you will see orange paints on nearby spruce trees. Nestled among the spruce trees and along Herlihy Road are campsites maintained by the Department of Environmental Conservation. Camping is by permit only, but permits can be obtained through the contact info provided on page 105. The trail briefly follows Herlihy Road before turning right, passing through a small section of spruce trees, and then joining Onondaga One Road. Bear right on this road and follow it briefly to where double orange paints mark the trail's entry back into the forest on the left.

The trail heads generally northeast and climbs gently. About 0.25 mile in, the trail crosses a snowmobile route and the trail grows steeper until you reach a left turn in the trail near the state forest boundary. In this section of the forest, long swaths of trees have been clear-cut. The narrow clear-cut strips create wide openings in the forest canopy, and carpets of ferns and other lush understory grow near and around these swaths. This adds a bit more diversity to the trail, and no doubt berry picking could be abundant at the right time of year.

After turning northward, the trail descends for a while before making a final ascent to Fellows Hill near the northern boundary of the state land. An ammo canister affixed to one of the spruce trees, typical for Finger Lakes Trail registers, marks the summit of the hill that some claim to be the highest point in Onondaga County, at 2,019 feet. A United States Geological Survey marker from 1934 can be found near the trail on a moss-covered stone. However, little else would let you know that you have reached a high point because the area is densely forested, without even a hint of a vista. From this high point, the trail continues westerly and declines 450 feet over the next 0.6 mile. By the time you reach Herlihy Road, you are actually 150 feet lower than when you began the approach to Fellows Hill from Onondaga One Road. Turn left and follow Herlihy Road about 1 mile back to the camping area beside Spruce Pond. Orange paints beside the road mark the return to the Spruce Pond campground, 4.5 miles overall. To finish, return 1.5 miles to Jones Hill and the hang glider launch point, and then descend 1 mile farther to the Tinker Falls Trailhead.

Directions

From the north: From the intersection of NY 80 and NY 91, just east of Apulia Station, turn onto NY 91 South/Apulia-Truxton Road. Head south 3.3 miles, past Labrador Cross Road and the Labrador Hollow Unique Area complex, to the large pulloff on the west side of the road.

From the south: From the intersection of NY 13 and NY 91 in Truxton, turn onto NY 91 North/Apulia-Truxton Road. Head north 5 miles to the large pulloff on the west side of the road.

13 # Carpenter's Falls Unique Area & Bahar Nature Preserve

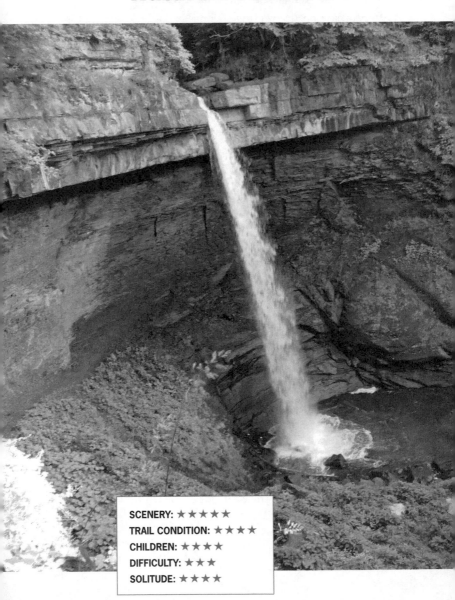

SCENERY: ★ ★ ★ ★ ★
TRAIL CONDITION: ★ ★ ★ ★
CHILDREN: ★ ★ ★ ★
DIFFICULTY: ★ ★ ★
SOLITUDE: ★ ★ ★ ★

GPS TRAILHEAD COORDINATES: N42° 48.8122'   W76° 20.4974'

DISTANCE & CONFIGURATION: 2.0-mile out-and-back; 0.3-mile side trip to Carpenter's Falls

HIKING TIME: 1.5–2 hours

HIGHLIGHTS: Spectacular waterfalls, scenic lake view

ELEVATION: 1,280' at trailhead; 866' at Skaneateles Lake shoreline

ACCESS: Open 24/7; no fees or permits required

MAPS: fllt.org (search for "Carpenter's Falls"); USGS *Spafford*

FACILITIES: None

WHEELCHAIR ACCESS: No

COMMENTS: The ravine surrounding the falls is very steep; use extreme caution when exploring the area.

CONTACTS: Finger Lakes Land Trust, 607-275-9487, **fllt.org/protected_lands /protected_lands1.php?id=33**; NYSDEC Region 7, 315-426-7400, **dec.ny.gov /outdoor/7792.html**

Overview

Certainly the main attraction here is the spectacular Carpenter's Falls. Nearly 90 feet tall, it is a beautiful example of a "hanging" falls, typical across the Finger Lakes region. Though the lakeside frontage is small, it makes a great destination and is another pretty feature adding variety to this trail.

Route Details

The trail described here crosses two different properties: the Carpenter's Falls Unique Area owned by the Department of Environmental Conservation (DEC) and the Bahar Nature Preserve owned by the Finger Lakes Lands Trust (FLLT). The acquisition of the 90 acres surrounding Bear Swamp Creek took more than a decade, starting with the original acquisition of 25 acres in 1998 from Hu Bahar, the preserve's namesake. In 2008 the FLLT transferred ownership of the land surrounding Carpenter's Falls to the DEC, but the FLLT still assists with stewardship of the area and trails. A common misconception is that parking is available on the lakeshore end of the trail, which is not

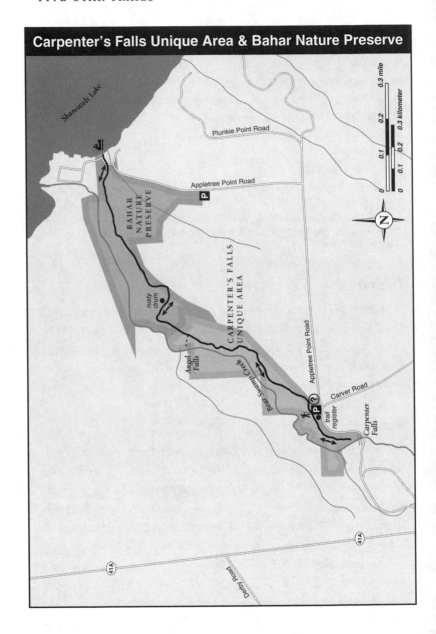

Carpenter's Falls Unique Area & Bahar Nature Preserve

true. Indeed parking at this end annoys local residents and will only increase friction between hikers and residents.

The parking area at the junction of Appletree Point and Carver Roads is suitable for a half dozen cars, and you will easily see the trailhead, kiosk, and register a few feet away. The kiosk is covered with numerous notices warning visitors that the ravines are steep, dangerous, and slippery and to stay on the trail. Though these types of notices are often ignored as no more than disclaimers, in this case hikers should pay attention. The ravines' sides are eroding due to heavy traffic and explorations, and we can only hope that someday the trails will be developed so that visitors can enjoy views of the falls without having to scramble about and erode the surrounding environment. To that end hikers should sign into the register, so the DEC knows that people use and enjoy the area. It is a simple way to let the DEC know to maintain and develop the area, so people can enjoy the trails conscientiously and safely.

The trail to Carpenter's Falls, marked by white paint, is to the left of the kiosk and follows a fairly broad stone-dust path. Follow the trail west 0.15 mile to a fork in the trail, where you can glimpse the falls through the surrounding forest. To the left is a path leading to the top of the falls, where Bear Swamp Creek has cut a path through the hard capstone. From this vantage point, you can look down onto

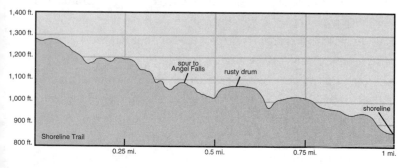

the gorge below. To the right is a myriad of paths that weave their way down the hillside to a view of the falls at the base.

Carpenter's Falls is categorized as a "hanging" falls and is truly a spectacular example. Hanging falls are formed when water flows over a hard, erosion-resistant capstone and then carves out softer stone beneath. The erosion often washes out behind the capstone, producing the effect of a shelf protruding far beyond the rock below. Approximately 90 feet high, Carpenter's Falls produces a spray and mist that allow moss and other verdant vegetation to grow in the amphitheater-like basin. At the base of the falls, the stones are slick with water and algae, so watch your footing. As noted, the hillside and base of the falls are composed of crumbly shale, so extra care should be taken when climbing to and from the base. No doubt you will want to take many pictures and linger in this scenic setting; plan on adding extra time to your trip to really enjoy this feature.

Return to the kiosk the way you came, and follow the main trail down to the lakeshore. The main trail to the shore, also marked with white paint, is a gradual descent of approximately 420 feet over 1 mile. The trail follows the southern rim of the gorge, and though you can hear Bear Swamp Creek, you will rarely see it off to your left. Approximately 0.3 mile from the kiosk, you catch a glimpse through the surrounding forest of one of several small falls along Bear Swamp Creek, but this one is inaccessible. As you continue, the tumble of water will grow louder, and eventually you can see the top of Angel Falls. Angel Falls is similar to Carpenter's Falls but is broader, has less of an overhang, and is 65 feet tall. A little farther along the trail, you will reach a point where many people have scrambled down into the gorge to reach the base of Angel Falls. In case you missed the warnings at the kiosk and throughout this description, the ravine sides are very steep. No kidding; that's why it is described as a ravine. In the current state of development, I can't recommend the very steep scramble down, but I hope someday an accessible trail will be provided so hikers can safely reach the base of Angel Falls.

Continuing along the main trail toward the shore of Skaneateles Lake, you pass beyond the boundaries of the DEC Carpenter's Falls Unique Area and into the Bahar Nature Preserve. Approximately 0.6 mile from the kiosk, you might notice a large rusty metal drum on your left. I'm not entirely sure, but this drum may be a remnant of the distilleries rumored to have existed along this creek. In the 1800s a trail from the lake led to gin mills atop Carpenter's Falls, and during the Prohibition era the forest and gorge were reported to provide excellent seclusion for parched boaters to follow the "Old Jug Path" for a private drink. Regardless, the drum marks a point approximately two-thirds of the way down to the lakeshore.

As you near the lakeshore, the trail begins to broaden enough for two to walk side by side, and you will be able to see the deep blue of Skaneateles Lake through the surrounding forest. The trail descends along a small creek to the right near its end at Appletree Point Road. Some people may choose to return along the road to the parking area to make a loop trip of 2.3 miles, but I prefer the solitude of the forest over hiking along a roadside. Across the road is a small grassy area that provides 65 feet of shoreline access. It's an ideal spot to take a short break before returning or a place for paddlers to pull up their boats before making an excursion up Old Jug Path and the falls.

Directions

From NY 20 in Skaneateles: Turn south onto NY 41A and follow it for 10.5 miles before turning left onto Appletree Point Road. Follow Appletree Point Road 0.5 mile to the intersection with Carver Road on your right. The parking area is on your left just before a dead-end sign.

From points south: Turn on NY 41A off of NY 41, and follow it 14.3 miles before turning right onto Appletree Point Road. This is 0.83 mile north of the intersection with CR 66A. Follow Appletree Point Road 0.5 mile to the intersection with Carver Road on your right. The parking area is on your left just before a dead-end sign.

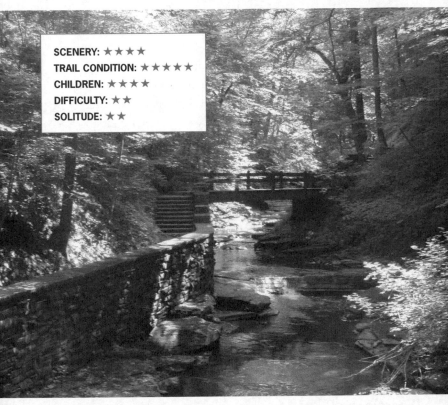

SCENERY: ★ ★ ★ ★
TRAIL CONDITION: ★ ★ ★ ★ ★
CHILDREN: ★ ★ ★ ★
DIFFICULTY: ★ ★
SOLITUDE: ★ ★

GPS TRAILHEAD COORDINATES: N42° 41.934'   W76° 24.980'

DISTANCE & CONFIGURATION: 2.5-mile out-and-back; 3.0-mile loop

HIKING TIME: 1–1.5 hours

HIGHLIGHTS: Waterfalls, scenic gorge

ELEVATION: 790' at trailhead, 1,182' at gorge rim

ACCESS: Daily, sunrise–sunset; Gorge Trail open only mid-May–November; $7 vehicle entrance fee

MAPS: nysparks.com/parks/157/maps.aspx; also available at entrance booth

FACILITIES: Restrooms, concessions, swimming area, picnic area, campground

WHEELCHAIR ACCESS: No

COMMENTS: The Gorge Trail opens in the spring, but only after safety inspections and required repairs are complete. Check with the park if you plan to visit in early spring.

CONTACTS: Fillmore Glen State Park, 315-497-0130, nysparks.com/parks/157/details.aspx

Overview

Fillmore Glen has much in common with the other gorge-centric state parks in the region, Buttermilk Falls (pages 157 and 164), Robert H. Treman (page 175), Taughannock Falls (pages 133 and 139), and Watkins Glen (page 194), all of which have a swimming area, camping, picturesque waterscapes, day-use facilities, and trails that wander through gorges and along their rims. And yet even with all their similarities, each park has its own character and charm. Here the distinctive character is a network of bridges that weave from bank to bank, all further enhanced by a bit more solitude. A little off the beaten path and farther north than the Ithaca area gorges, this park sees fewer visitors but is still close enough to its brethren that the ambitious hiker could take in several gorges in one day.

Route Details

To reach the trailhead, walk through or around the large main pavilion and past the swimming and day-use area to the large wooden trail signs. Over the stone bridge on the left is the base of Cow Sheds waterfall as well as the return from the North Rim Trail. To the right, stairs lead up to the second day-use area and the Gorge Trail. The trail to the base of Cow Sheds is very short and often as far as some park visitors will go. Washing into a rubble-strewn stone amphitheater, it's an impressive falls that seems far taller than its 37 feet. No matter which route you choose to explore the park, all the trails lead back to this point, so you can view the Cow Sheds either at the start or conclusion of your trip. Like many of the state park gorge trails, you first have to head up and around the lower falls to reach the Gorge Trail.

Turn right and head up the worn steps. Once you reach the top, bear left and follow the asphalt path into the woods. If you choose to return via the southern rim, this collection of picnic tables and shelters is the point you would return to. The trail soon reaches a set of stone stairs that lead to a lookout above Cow Sheds Falls. No doubt you will hear the surge of water as it tumbles into the amphitheater

Fillmore Glen State Park

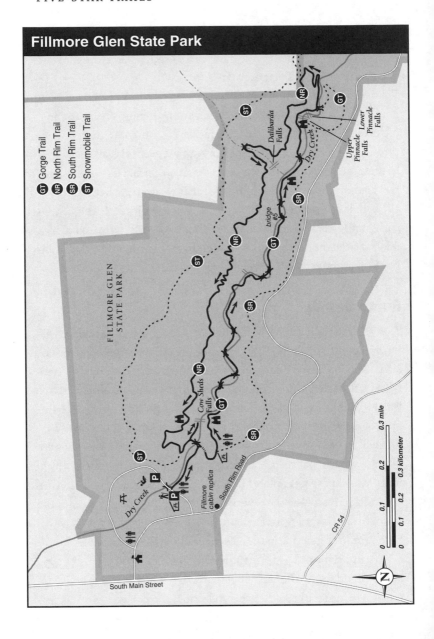

below, but the only section visible is the slightly obscured crest of the falls. Atop the falls, the stream is mostly flat and smooth, with occasional square cuts that form tiny flumes or short falls. The trail weaves to either side of the stream and crosses multiple bridges, the first of which is roughly 0.4 mile along. The next three bridges come in quick succession, and soon the trail is again on the southern side of the gorge. Mostly flat and lined with handsome stone walls, this next section is a pleasant stroll almost due east 0.25 mile. As you approach a sharp right turn in the trail, you will no doubt hear the crash of water ahead. A small falls with a tiny flume above is just around the turn in the gorge. Many worn paths lead down to the streambed and the falls' base, but those near the falls are heavily eroded, and the easiest way to navigate down is back along the trail before you reach the bend.

Back along the trail, the path briefly heads southward before swinging eastward as it climbs above the streambed. Recently added wood bridges carry you over a series of feeder streamlets; these are not to be confused with the main numbered bridges that span the gorge stream. The most handsome of these main bridges, bridge five, is just ahead at 0.9 mile where a wooden bridge crosses to a stone-walled landing on the northern shore. Walking along the stone landing feels a bit like walking the battlements above a surging moat. It's

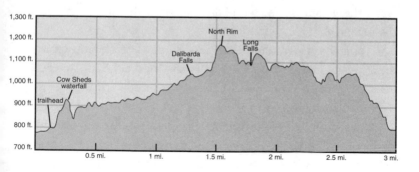

an iconic scene for the park and soon concludes after crossing the sixth bridge.

Shortly ahead is another sharp right turn along the trail and the second of the major falls, Dalibarda Falls, found within the gorge. To the left is a long cascade that, depending on the time of year, could be either a barely discernible veil falls or a frothy torrent. In summer, the understory and overarching trees mask how truly tall these falls are, but in autumn you can see that these are indeed the tallest of the falls in the gorge, at 85 feet.

Shortly ahead, bridge seven brings you back to the north side of the gorge and to a stone-scaped walk that leads to the final major falls along Fillmore Creek, sometimes called Dry Creek. Stone pillars with log rails line the gorge side of the trail, while a series of square-cut alcoves are found periodically on the left. As you come around one of these oddly uniform alcoves, a wide square-cut falls, Lower Pinnacle Falls, looms ahead. Stone stairs take you down to a U-shaped viewing area along the path and then back up to where the trail winds southward around to the top of these 25-foot-tall falls. Stone-scaping and more alcoves line the path here. Don't forget to look back downstream to take in the full scope of the scene as you near the final waterfall along the trail. The smaller square-cut Upper Pinnacle Falls marks the end of the gorge, the waterscapes, and in effect the Gorge Trail. The eighth bridge is located here and leads across the stream to the South Rim Trail, while the North Rim Trail lies straight ahead.

As is the case with most gorge trails, you have a choice: Return the way you came or follow a rim trail back. The South Rim Trail features the Pinnacle Overlook, but the view is mostly obscured, especially in the summer when the foliage is full. The rest of the path along the South Rim offers little variety and basically follows a park road most of the way. While not entirely scenic, the North Rim does follow mostly a woodland path, and it visits the top of the Dalibarda Falls. Additionally, near the North Rim's conclusion there are some masked views of Cow Sheds waterfall. Of the three I would say the

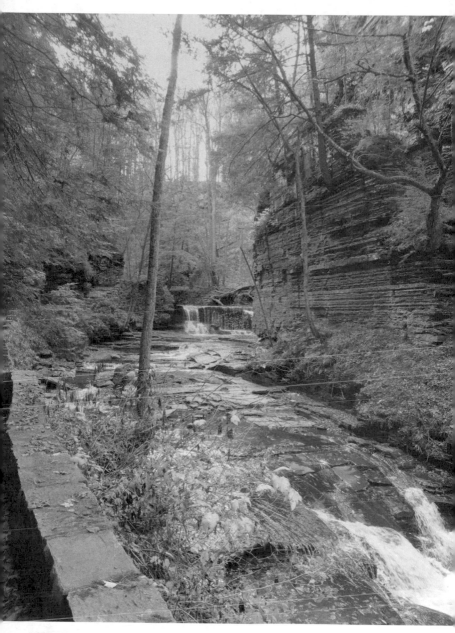

LAST FALLS

North Rim is my recommended return route because it also adds a bit of solitude, as most hikers remain along the Gorge Trail.

To reach the North Rim, continue straight and soon reach a series of steep switchbacks that climb 150 feet in less than 0.25 mile. At the top, you reach a trail sign noting that the North Rim also continues east to the dam at the eastern edge of the park. Turn left and begin the mostly downhill trek back to the lower park. You reach the top of the Dalibarda Falls in about 0.25 mile (1.66 miles overall). Unfortunately the banks are too narrow and steep to see much of the falls from up here, but the walk beside its source is a pleasant change of pace for an otherwise featureless return trip along the rim. At around 2.5 miles, traverse a steeper portion of the descent back, and near its conclusion Cow Sheds Falls can be heard and seen off to the left. At the bottom, turn left and head back to the arched stone bridge and visit (or revisit) Cow Sheds before you return to the parking area, for an overall trip length of 2.8 miles.

Directions

From I-81, take Exit 12 (US 11/NY 41/NY 2181) toward Homer/Cortland. Follow the off-ramp to the traffic light, and turn right on South West Street. After 0.4 mile, turn left onto NY 90 North/Cayuga Street and follow it 12.8 miles. Turn right onto NY 38 North/Main Street, go 2.8 miles, and the park entrance is on the right.

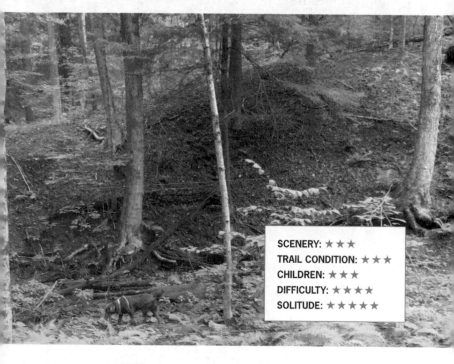

SCENERY: ★ ★ ★
TRAIL CONDITION: ★ ★ ★
CHILDREN: ★ ★ ★
DIFFICULTY: ★ ★ ★ ★
SOLITUDE: ★ ★ ★ ★ ★

GPS TRAILHEAD COORDINATES: N42° 40.007'   W75° 54.378'

DISTANCE & CONFIGURATION: 4.6-mile point to point; 3.0-mile out-and-back side trip to Chippewa Falls; loop options described below

HIKING TIME: 2.5–3.5 hours

HIGHLIGHTS: Waterfall, quiet woodland, secluded glen

ELEVATION: 1,820' at trailhead; 2,080' at highest point along trail

ACCESS: Open 24/7; no fees or permits required

MAPS: DEC Cuyler Hill State Forest map: **dec.ny.gov/lands/37269.html**; Finger Lakes Trail Conference: Sheet M21

FACILITIES: None

WHEELCHAIR ACCESS: No

COMMENTS: Plan on using two vehicles or catching a lift for this point-to-point trek. Otherwise, the trail length is 9.2 miles. Alternatively you can return along forest roads for a less strenuous 8.2-mile loop. Remember to add 3 miles to your trip planning if you include Chippewa Falls. Also note that Potter Hill Cemetery Road is not plowed in the winter.

CONTACTS: NYSDEC Region 7, Cortland Sub-Office, 607-753-3095, **dec.ny.gov /lands/37028.html**

Cuyler Hill State Forest

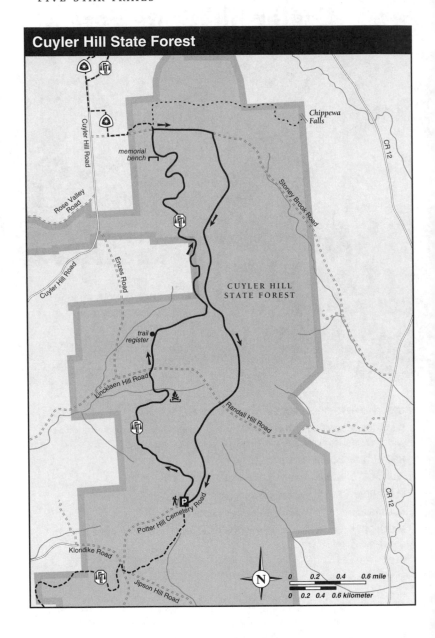

Chippewa Falls

memorial bench

Cuyler Hill Road

Rose Valley Road

Cuyler Hill Road

Enzes Road

Stoney Brook Road

CR 12

CUYLER HILL STATE FOREST

trail register

Lincklaen Hill Road

Randall Hill Road

CR 12

Potter Hill Cemetery Road

Klondike Road

Jipson Hill Road

N

0   0.2   0.4   0.6 mile

0   0.2   0.4   0.6 kilometer

Overview

Much of the rolling terrain in Cuyler Hill State Forest passes through extensive tree planting by Civilian Conservation Corps (CCC) crews from the 1930s. Varied terrain, seasonal streams, and different forest types provide ample variety along this end-to-end trek. Changes in elevation mean a more strenuous trip than you'll find on the otherwise flat trails in the region, and options for extending your hike offer an additional challenge. During the spring melt, a side trip to Chippewa Falls is recommended, but be aware that its path is overgrown and the falls run dry during the summer.

Route Details

Before beginning your trip to Cuyler Hill State Forest, you need to plan your strategy. The trail described below is end to end and requires either two cars or being shuttled from one end to the other. Don't expect to catch a lift, as the roads are rarely traveled. Or you can employ a hike-and-bike strategy, where you leave a bike at one end of the trail and park your car at the other end. This strategy might not work well along many trails, but in the Cuyler Hill State Forest a rugged access road roughly follows the trail. This road is described in the trail directions following and could make an interesting ride. Alternatively you could hike this road to form a less strenuous loop

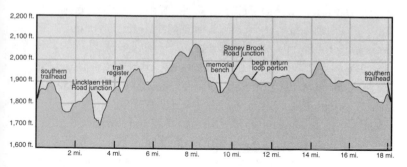

than if you choose to hike the trail as an out-and-back. Finally, a side trip of 1.5 miles to Chippewa Falls (3 miles total) is located near the main trail's conclusion. Account for additional time and energy if you include it in your trip.

Parking for the southern trailhead is about 0.1 mile north of where the Finger Lakes Trail (FLT) crosses Potter Hill Cemetery Road. While the parking is hard to discern along the dirt road, the FLT markers on either side of the road are highly visible. Begin the trail on the north side of the road, following white FLT blazes. As you make your way north, you'll notice that the forest fluctuates between hardwood and softwood. The variety is a result of extensive tree plantings that took place in the 1930s. In an effort to counteract the continued erosion by poor farming practices, nearly 2.5 million trees were planted by two different CCC camps. Later, an additional half million trees were planted by the Department of Environmental Conservation. Today stands of northern hardwoods, spruces, pines, cedars, and hemlocks dot the landscape, and you will pass through many of these different forest covers.

After a short initial climb and descent, the beginning portion of the trail follows a relatively level sweeping arc northwest around the contours of one of several knobs along Randall Hill. At roughly 1.25 miles, you begin a steep 160-foot descent into Wiltsley Glen. At the bottom of the descent, the trail turns sharply westward and parallels the stream within this secluded glen. Off to the right is a bivouac area with a small stone fire pit situated beside the stream. No doubt thru-hikers along the 562-mile FLT find this an appealing stop.

The trail continues a short way westward before crossing the seasonal stream and beginning a 200-foot climb. A little over halfway along the climb, the trail intersects Randall Hill Road; some maps note this as Lincklaen Hill Road. Cross the road and continue to climb along the contours of the second of Randall Hill's knobs, Accordion Summit. Pass a green-painted ammo can affixed to a tree, repurposed as an FLT register, at 1.8 miles. Nearby is an orange-marked trail that descends to another bivouac area, Rose Hollow. Past this point the trail follows an easterly course for about 0.5 mile before swinging north again. After a short descent, you'll begin a long, steady climb of 220 feet to the highest point along Randall Hill, at 2,080 feet. Along this 1.25-mile stretch are numerous wet areas, and as you follow the contours of this ridge, you may even catch a few glimpses of the opposing valley to the west. When leafed out, the scene is obscured, but fall and winter promise a more scenic perspective. The "summit" is amid dense forest, so don't expect grand vistas, and as soon as you reach the top, you begin a steep descent. A series of switchbacks brings you 0.4 mile ahead and 250 feet down to a washed-out delta along another seasonal stream. You briefly weave along the south bank of this stream before switching back and following its north bank westward, where a memorial bench provides a resting spot. The bench is dedicated to Randall E. Brune, who designed and built the trail. From here it is another 0.25 mile to the trail's end at Stoney Brook Road (4.6 miles overall).

From here, pick up your shuttle car, or proceed (by foot or by bike) along a loop using forest roads as follows: Travel along Stoney Brook Road east for 0.4 mile; then take your first right and follow Cortland Six Road 2.3 miles to Randall Hill Road. Cross Randall Hill Road and follow Potter Hill Cemetery Road 0.9 mile south to your vehicle.

However, if you visit in the spring or after heavy rains, it might be worth making the short trek to Chippewa Falls. To reach the falls, continue across the road, now following blue blazes. The route forward used to be part of the FLT, but when private-property owners decided to no longer allow access through their property, the trail had to be rerouted eastward. The North Country Trail (NCT) continues north along the Onondaga Trail, which continues a short way into the forest to a trail junction. The NCT and Onondaga Trail depart on your left, while straight, marked in orange, is the path to Chippewa Falls. Shortly after the intersection, the trail swings east and follows a gentle decline and then rises over the next 0.5 mile. Now that it is no longer a part of the FLT, the path is lightly traveled, and brush and brambles become dense along some sections. Gaiters are advised during the summer. You reach the crest of this short climb about 0.75 mile along the trail and begin the final winding descent to the falls. Along the descent you will pass close to the state forest's northern edge, where roofs and buildings become briefly visible on your left. You reach the creek that feeds the falls in a small hemlock grove shortly before you near the crest of the falls.

Chippewa Falls is often dry, but during the spring it surges as it falls dozens of feet over a steep rock wall. One waterfall guidebook estimates the falls' total drop to more than 200 feet, but this must include lower sections not visible from the upper viewing area. It's tempting to try to get lower to view the falls, but the terrain is very steep and soon passes into private property, so venturing farther is not only unwise but prohibited. Seen from the side, the falls are still impressive, and the grove of hemlocks creates a primeval scene distinct from other sections of the trail. Return 1.5 miles to Stoney Brook Road for a trip length of 7.6 miles.

Directions

From NY 13/Main Street in Cuyler, turn onto CR 152B/Tripoli Road. At 0.1 mile, continue straight onto CR 152A/Lincklaen Hill Road. Turn right onto Cuyler Hill Road at 1.9 miles. Follow Cuyler Hill Road for 1.5 miles, and turn right onto Stoney Brook Road. The end of the northern trailhead is 0.5 mile ahead on your right. Leave your first car or bike here and continue 0.4 mile; take the first right onto Cortland Six Road (unmarked). Cross Randall Hill Road at 2.3 miles, and continue straight onto Potter Hill Cemetery Road (unmarked). Follow Potter Hill Cemetery Road 0.9 mile south, where a small pulloff is located on the east side of the road. The trailhead is 0.1 mile farther down the road on your right.

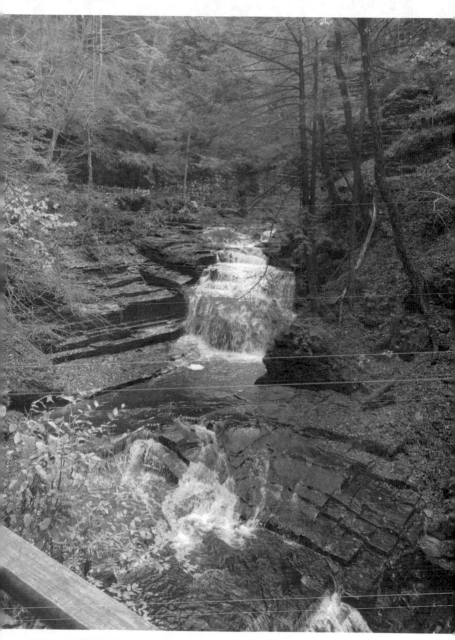

TRAIL 14 UPPER FALLS AT FILLMORE GLEN STATE PARK *see page 116*

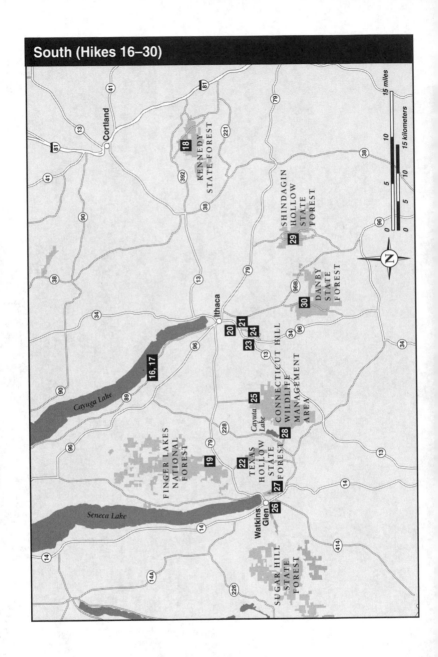

South

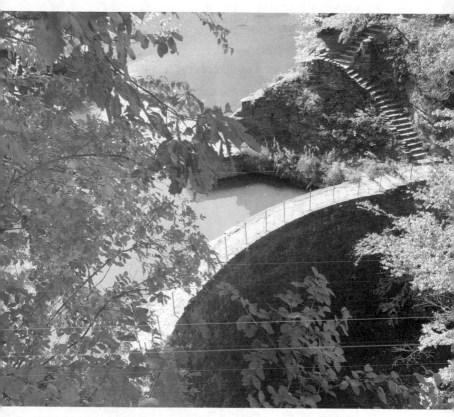

TRAIL 21 BUTTERMILK FALLS STATE PARK: LAKE TREMAN LOOP
see page 164

Continued on next page

Taughannock Falls
State Park: Gorge Trail

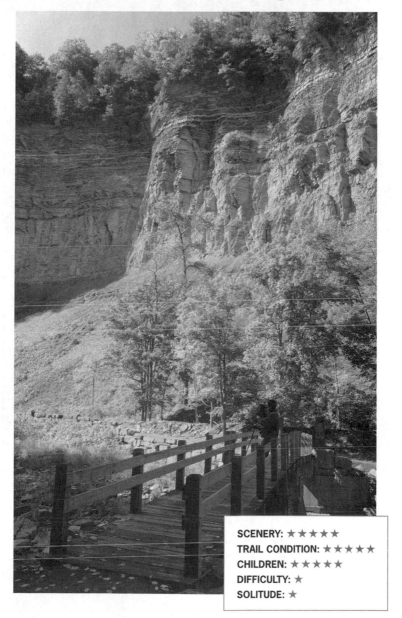

SCENERY: ★ ★ ★ ★ ★
TRAIL CONDITION: ★ ★ ★ ★ ★
CHILDREN: ★ ★ ★ ★ ★
DIFFICULTY: ★
SOLITUDE: ★

Taughannock Falls State Park: Gorge Trail

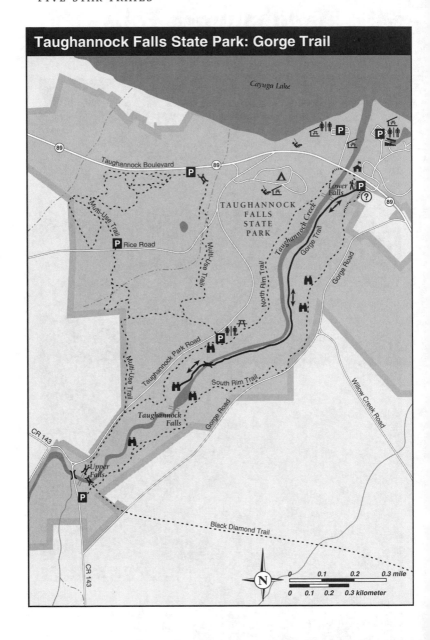

GPS TRAILHEAD COORDINATES: N42° 32.734'   W76° 35.962'

DISTANCE & CONFIGURATION: 1.5-mile out-and-back

HIKING TIME: 1 hour

HIGHLIGHTS: Waterfalls, scenic gorge

ELEVATION: 405' at trailhead, with no significant rise

ACCESS: Daily, sunrise–sunset; $7 vehicle entrance fee

MAPS: nysparks.com/parks/62/maps.aspx; also available at entrance booth

FACILITIES: Restrooms, concessions, swimming area, picnic area, campground

WHEELCHAIR ACCESS: Yes (Gorge Trail only)

COMMENTS: The Gorge Trail is a popular destination, so plan your trip in off-seasons and/or during the week to avoid the crowds.

CONTACTS: Taughannock Falls State Park, 607-387-6739, **nysparks.com/parks/62/details.aspx**

Overview

More accurately described as a canyon, the gorge at Taughannock Falls State Park is immense. The falls are 215 feet tall, 31 feet taller than Niagara Falls, and are considered the tallest free-falling waterfall east of the Rockies. The flat trail to the base of the falls is easily accessible for all.

Route Details

The trails in the park consist of two separate trips: the 1.5-mile out-and-back Gorge Trail described here and the 2.8-mile Rim Trail, detailed beginning on page 139. Unlike other gorge trails at nearby state parks, where gorge and rim trails form a loop, the two at Taughannock Falls are not connected. Furthermore, I can't recommend one over the other. Instead, I suggest that you hike both. For the most dramatic perspective, hike the Gorge Trail first, so that later when you look down on your previous path, you can take in the true depth of this canyon.

To accurately describe what you should expect, perhaps it would be helpful to differentiate between some common terms used to describe gorges: canyons, ravines, and gullies. All are considered gorges, with the main difference being a matter of magnitude. Gorges have steep walls and are narrower than valleys. Gullies are the smallest, though ditches are also considered lesser members of this topographical category. Ravines lie in between, while canyons are the largest of the group.

The Gorge Trail is perhaps one of the easiest trails featured in this book. It is also one of the most popular among tourists, so don't expect privacy. However, the falls and the broad canyon are both stunning and worth joining the crowds for a little while. The trail follows what is essentially a flat road, roughly 8–10 feet wide, 0.75 mile to the base of the falls. During the summer and on weekends, there are lots of visitors, but thankfully the broad trail means that at least the path won't be congested and you are free to move at your desired pace. Directions along the trail are unnecessary, so a synopsis of what to expect will suffice. The first point of interest is the Lower Falls, a 15-foot cascade that faces a large lawn and picnic area beside the parking area on the west side of NY 89. Past this waterfall is a small hill, barely a few feet high and perhaps the only real ascent along this trail. From this point forward you will walk along essentially level ground at the base of the broad canyon. The sheer cliff walls that encompass the gorge are almost 400 feet tall. Taughannock Creek has a nearly flat, broad limestone bed that at times looks more like a flooded paved highway than a creek. Nearly square-cut ledges along the creek bed provide some cascades, but don't expect the dramatic waterscapes found along other gorge trails. During the summer large portions of the creek bed are dry and often filled with hikers, ignoring the "stay on designated trails" warnings.

Many people choose to stroll along this flat trail, but hikers who enjoy a vigorous pace will find themselves at the wood bridge at the base of the falls in practically no time whatsoever. Although the trail thus far has offered many sights of the sheer cliff walls, coming out into the amphitheater-like basin that surrounds the base of the falls is truly amazing. The falls drop 215 feet into a 30-foot-deep plunge pool, though for safety's sake the trail ends well away from the pool. Exploring the base of the falls, including swimming, is

MOVIE MAGIC

Think that this canyon would make a dramatic scene for a movie? Well, early in the 20th century, many people agreed. For a brief time, Ithaca was considered the center of the budding movie industry. Silent films were just beginning, and filmmakers found that Ithaca's beautiful gorges and natural landscapes were a perfect setting for their cliff-hanger serials. Eventually Hollywood became the center of film production, but Ithaca was in the running to be the film capital of the United States, if only for a short while.

strictly prohibited. The basin is actively eroding, with large chunks of rocks, sometimes as big as a house, falling into the basin below. In 2005 a woman was killed and three others injured by one of these rockslides. In 2010 a 54-foot-wide boulder was documented falling into the basin. Dramatic before-and-after photos of this rockslide are available at **nyfalls.com/taughannock-rock-fall.html.**

Taughannock Falls is a beautiful example of a hanging valley. During the Pleistocene epoch, which began more than 2 million years ago, the preexisting Cayuga River Valley was scoured deeply by immense sheets of ice. Indeed the bulldozing of Cayuga Lake has left its bottom 36 feet below sea level. Glaciers receded and advanced over thousands of years, but its final advance and retreat, known as the Wisconsinan Phase, ended in New York approximately 12,000 years ago. When a glacier halts in its advance or stalls in its retreat, it deposits great masses of unsorted materials into moraines. The Head Valley Moraine is one such example, and it extends in an erratic arc along the southern edge of the Finger Lakes. In some circumstances the moraine created dams, halting the flow of water south, the predominant direction of the flow of rivers before glaciation began. When the retreat continued, meltwater became trapped between the moraine and ice, creating immense lakes. When the ice retreated further, lake levels dropped and the streams and valleys that once fed the lake were left "hanging" above. Progressively, water flowing over the hanging valley cut back into the newly created cliff face, slowly elongating the gorge. At Taughannock Falls, this dramatic erosion is enhanced by the fact that the gorge is composed of layers of rock with varying erosion resistance. In this circumstance, the creek within the lower gorge flows over hard and very erosion-resistant Tully Limestone, while the walls are composed of hundreds of feet of crumbly Geneseo Shale. At the crest of the falls, the creek flows over erosion-resistant Sherburne Sandstone and continues to undercut and erode the shale in between these two resistant layers. Although the capstone is erosion resistant, it is not as resistant as those capstones found at Tinker Falls (page 98) or Carpenter's Falls (page 110). At those waterfalls the capstones are so resistant to wear that they extend out into the air, providing an overhang and carved-out amphitheater behind the falls. Here, the capstone frequently falls away and the gorge elongates at a faster pace. Over thousands of years the shale is washed away and deposited into the broad delta along Cayuga Lake that serves as the day-use area at the park. For a more in-depth perspective on this process, head back to the trailhead and begin the Rim Trail, described on the following pages.

Directions

From most points east and south: From Ithaca, head north along NY 89. Follow NY 89 on the east side of Cayuga Lake 9.3 miles to the trail parking area on your left.

From most points west and north: Take Exit 41 along the New State Thruway, I-90. Merge onto NY 414 South, and turn left onto NY 318 East. After 1.1 miles, turn left on NY 5/NY 20/Auburn Road, and immediately turn right onto NY 89 South. Follow NY 89 South 32 miles past Taughannock Park Road to the trail parking area on your right.

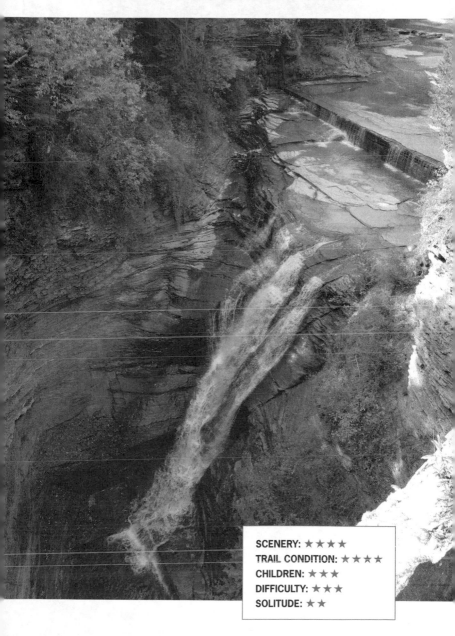

SCENERY: ★ ★ ★ ★
TRAIL CONDITION: ★ ★ ★ ★
CHILDREN: ★ ★ ★
DIFFICULTY: ★ ★ ★
SOLITUDE: ★ ★

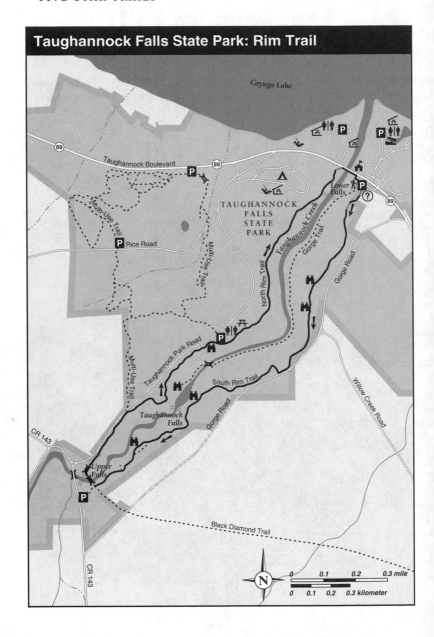

Taughannock Falls State Park: Rim Trail

GPS TRAILHEAD COORDINATES: N42° 32.734'   W76° 35.962'

DISTANCE & CONFIGURATION: 2.8-mile loop

HIKING TIME: 1–2 hours

HIGHLIGHTS: Waterfalls, scenic gorge, panoramic vistas

ELEVATION: 405' at trailhead; 830' at highest point along Rim Trail

ACCESS: Daily, sunrise–sunset (sections of the Rim Trail are closed for the winter);
$7 vehicle entrance fee

MAPS: nysparks.com/parks/62/maps.aspx; also available at entrance booth

FACILITIES: Restrooms, concessions, swimming area, picnic area, campground

WHEELCHAIR ACCESS: No

COMMENTS: Sections of the Rim Trail are closed during the winter, but alternative routes
are available. Call ahead to plan your trip.

CONTACTS: Taughannock Falls State Park, 607-387-6739, **nysparks.com/parks/62**
/details.aspx

Overview

The trail into the scenic Taughannock Falls gorge is not the only spectacular trail within the park. Unlike many rim trails at other state
parks, the rim trail here is full of scenic vistas into the canyon below,
views of the towering 215-foot Taughannock Falls and the 80-foot
Upper Falls, and a panoramic perspective of Cayuga Lake as well. I
recommend that you hike the rim in the clockwise direction, as it
puts the least scenic section at the beginning and allows for even better views of the lake while you descend to the trailhead.

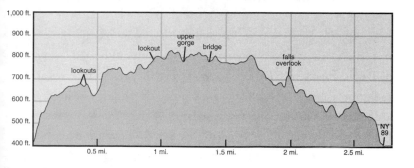

Route Details

The Rim Trail begins to the left of the sign and kiosk at the beginning of the Gorge Trail (see page 133). The trail quickly climbs 150 feet in a little over 0.1 mile along a series of stairs. Once past the stairs, the trail begins to level off, though you'll experience a definite slight incline as you make your way approximately 1.3 miles to the bridge that separates the South Rim and North Rim sections. Approximately 0.3 mile along the South Rim Trail, you pass the first of several small lookouts that provide interesting views of the canyon below. A handful of these undesignated lookouts are along both the southern and northern rims. Often these lookouts are just small openings in the lower canopy, providing leaf-framed views. These "windowed" views are limited in the summer, but in fall after the leaves are gone, you can imagine an entirely new perspective of the canyon. Regardless of the time of visit, the vistas are serene and yet also stunning when you compare the steep shale cliffs to the tiny dots (that is, hikers) along the canyon floor. Another fine scenic spot is a short distance ahead, where the trail comes into view of Gorge Road on your left. The Rim Trail is heavily forested, but much of the path lies within earshot and even sight of public roads, unfortunately spoiling any wilderness atmosphere. Indeed a short distance farther, the trail joins the road, if only briefly, and then heads back into the park near a sign labeled "South Rim."

Approximately 1 mile in from the beginning of the rim circuit, you reach another unmarked lookout. You can hear the surge of Taughannock Falls down to your left, but the falls themselves are sadly not visible. Instead what draws your eye is the tiny viewing area at the base of the falls. Spacious and large when you were previously down there shooting photos upward, the end of the trail and tiny hikers now appear small and insignificant. You are, of course, 400 feet above them, and I do not recommend this sight downward to those who tend to get a touch of vertigo.

Continue southeast another 0.3 mile and you emerge from the forest onto an open bedrock shelf. Lined with chain-link fences, this tableau sits above the upper canyon along Taughannock Creek. This is the first lookout designated on the park map. Several benches here prove a pleasant stopping point for those who wish to bask in the sun. Below is a much narrower and wilder gorge than the canyon previously seen. A small square-shaped falls tumbles a little farther up the path and just below a small lookout that protrudes into the gorge. It doesn't take a stretch of imagination to envision that the canyon behind once looked very much like this upper gorge. It took 10,000–12,000 years for the crest of Taughannock Falls to recede back approximately 1 mile. How much longer before this upper section is washed away as well?

A very short distance farther, you come into sight of an old railroad bridge built with deep steel girders. You will pass under this bridge shortly and reach an intersection. Ahead is the upper parking area, while back and to your left are steps that lead to the top of the bridge and the path across Taughannock Creek to the North Rim Trail. I hardly have to advise you to look to your left (west) while you cross the bridge because the roar of the Upper Falls will have drawn your attention already. Nearly 80 foot tall, the Upper Falls are a beautiful sight in their own right. A tiny bit upstream you glimpse a handsome stone bridge along Jacksonville Road. After taking your photos of the Upper Falls, don't forget to admire the scene of the upper gorge to the east. Practically speaking, this is the only vantage point where you are above and in the middle of the gorge.

Across the bridge a sign indicates that the North Rim Trail continues to your right. At this point you might notice a worn footpath that weaves its way under the bridge. This path takes you to another vantage point of the Upper Falls, but it's not nearly as interesting or as good as the view from the bridge. Continue northeast along a heavily worn footpath. You travel within clear sight of Taughannock Park Road about 0.25 mile to where the trail veers right into the forest. Along the next 0.5 mile to the Falls Overlook, there will be several

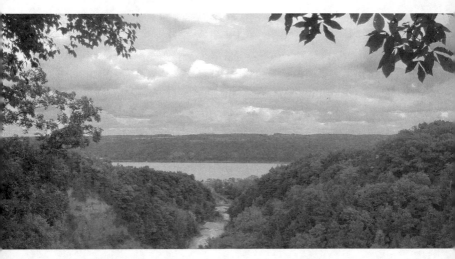

CAYUGA LAKE

decent "windowed" views of the main falls. When leaves are present, the base of the falls lies just out of sight of these portals, but the top of the falls is pleasantly framed. To see the falls in their entirety, you will have to join the throngs of visitors at the Falls Overlook.

The overlook has restrooms, and the parking area is typically filled to capacity during the summer and on weekends. To reach the overlook, you descend a series of stone stairs to a viewing platform. This is the spot where most pictures of the falls are taken. A word of warning: Visitors and hikers are not the only ones who congest the area. If you happen to visit on a summer weekend, then more than likely you will have to take your turn with—wait for it—weddings. Yes, the picturesque and dramatic overlook is a popular spot for wedding parties not only to take photos but also to hold ceremonies. So if the presence of cars is not enough to pull you out of your wilderness bliss, then I am sure the sudden appearance of ladies and gentlemen in full formal attire will be.

Back along the trail, head past the picnic area and you will soon pass a fenced-in research station. The purpose of the enclosure is to measure the difference between forests' growth when deer are removed from the equation. From this point forward, the trail begins a gradual descent to the trailhead. Along this descent several small undesignated lookouts provide even more peeks of the canyon below, but also some very scenic vistas of the canyon, its broad delta, and Cayuga Lake to the east. Few trails in the Finger Lakes provide comparable panoramic vistas of the region's lakes. The addition of lake scenery makes this rim loop even more noteworthy in my opinion.

You will pass by the back side of the park's campground at 2.6 miles. For a detailed description of the campgrounds, see *Best Tent Camping: New York State*. Just past the campground, you reach a steep set of stone stairs that lead down to NY 89. Bear right at the road, and head over the bridge back to the parking area for a round-trip of just under 3 miles, or 4.5 miles if you include the out-and-back to the base of the falls.

Nearby Attractions

One reason weddings are popular at the lookout is that many bed-and-breakfasts and wineries are found throughout the region and especially along NY 89. A full description of the wine trails is beyond the scope of this book, but planning a visit to at least one of the many renowned area wineries would likely enhance your trip.

Directions

From most points east and south: From Ithaca, head north along NY 89. Follow NY 89 on the east side of Cayuga Lake 9.3 miles to the trail parking area on your left.

From most points west and north: Take Exit 41 along the New State Thruway, I-90. Merge onto NY 414 South, and turn left onto NY 318 East. After 1.1 miles, turn left on NY 5/NY 20/Auburn Road, and immediately turn right onto NY 89 South. Follow NY 89 South 32 miles past Taughannock Park Road to the trail parking area on your right.

Virgil Mountain

18

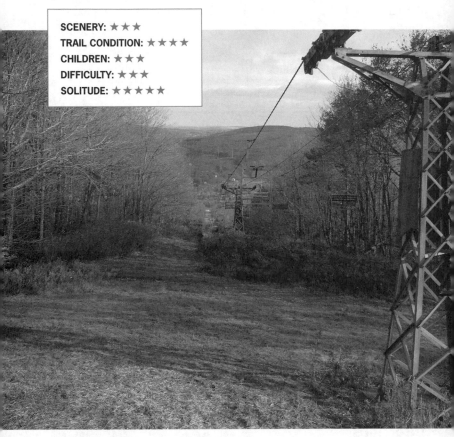

SCENERY: ★ ★ ★
TRAIL CONDITION: ★ ★ ★ ★
CHILDREN: ★ ★ ★
DIFFICULTY: ★ ★ ★
SOLITUDE: ★ ★ ★ ★ ★

GPS TRAILHEAD COORDINATES: N42° 29.250'   W76° 09.685'

DISTANCE & CONFIGURATION: 4.8-mile loop

HIKING TIME: 2 hours

HIGHLIGHTS: Quiet woodland, secluded glen, vista

ELEVATION: 1,724' at trailhead; 2,122' at highest point along trail

ACCESS: Open 24/7; no fees or permits required

MAPS: DEC James Kennedy State Forest area map: **dec.ny.gov/lands/9279.html**; Finger Lakes Trail Conference: Virgil Mt. Area Loops & Sheet M19

FACILITIES: None

WHEELCHAIR ACCESS: No

COMMENTS: In 2013 some sections were being rerouted, so be aware that trail paints may mark an old route and directions that follow may differ slightly from the final course trail builders chose. Old sections of the trail were still marked in white, but logs and debris were laid across the trail, and orange flags tied to saplings marked the new route. Regardless, the detours were brief and eventually reconnected with the old Finger Lakes Trail with insignificant differences in mileage.

CONTACTS: NYSDEC Region 7, Cortland Sub-Office, 607-753-3095, **dec.ny.gov** **/lands/8192.html**

Overview

Despite the misleading moniker of the trail, there are no mountains in Central New York. Rather, the landscape is dotted with forested, oversteepened hills, the vestiges of an ancient seabed upturned by a continental collision and then sculpted by massive ice sheets. Nearly uniform in character and practically the same height, these odd hilltops are everywhere in the Finger Lakes and Central New York. The trail here climbs to the top of two of these hills, and, unlike on many other hilltops in the region, here you are rewarded with a couple of vistas that reveal how uniform these hilltops are.

Route Details

The parking area is a small pulloff at the intersections of Odell and Baldwin Roads. From this pulloff, head north and uphill along Odell Road about 0.25 mile to where the Finger Lakes Trail (FLT) reenters the forest. Double white paints on the west side of the road and a yellow FLT sign on the right mark the entry point. Turn right and head east, crossing several small streams as you weave slightly uphill. The climb becomes steeper after the trail crosses a narrow stream with a rock wall visible uphill and to the left. From this point it is a 250-foot climb over the next 0.5 mile to the top of Greek Peak. The trail intersects Van Donsel Road about midway through this climb, at roughly the 1-mile marker. The trail passes by the ski lift at the top of Greek Peak, 2,098 feet, to the left. Some views of the landscape to the north are available near the lift, but more expansive views are found near the power lines that cross Virgil Mountain a little less than a mile ahead.

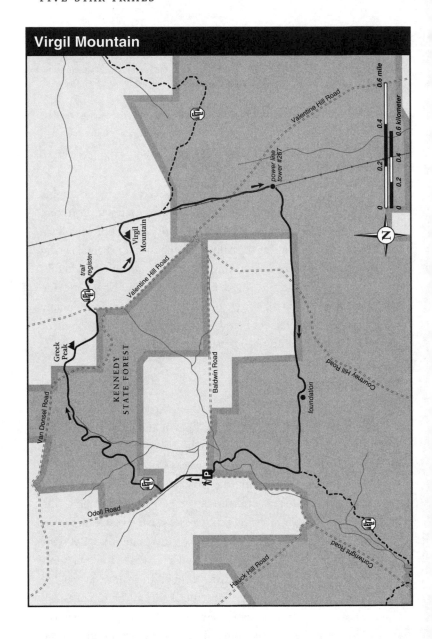

Virgil Mountain

The trail parallels an eastbound ski run as it weaves down into the notch between the two high points. Although they are the highest points in Cortland County, to call them mountains in anything but name seems a bit of a stretch. Near the belly of the notch, you pass a trail register at 1.8 miles. The trail swings southward at this point and begins a roughly 150-foot climb to Virgil Mountain. As you ascend the contours of the western edge of the hill, views of the opposing ridge are glimpsed through the forest to your right, especially after the leaves have fallen in autumn. Shortly after the trail curves due east, you reach the peak of Virgil Mountain (2,132 feet), a grassy hilltop encircled by forest with no views in any direction. However, if you continue east, you reach an access road and high-voltage power lines whose cut through the forest provides dramatic and panoramic views to the east and slightly to the north.

Turn right and follow the access road south. White paints can be seen on some of the stones within the road and occasionally on the power line towers. Just shy of 0.25 mile south along this road, the FLT departs to the left as it heads northeast to Tuller Hill State Forest. The turn is easy to miss, especially coming from this direction, but once the paints along the road have changed from white to orange, you'll know you have passed it. Continue heading south along the road past the intersection with Valentine Hill Road 0.3 mile ahead (2.7 miles

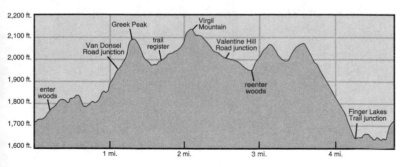

overall). About 0.25 mile past Valentine Hill Road, the access road jogs slightly near one of the high-voltage towers (number 267). Double orange paints and an arrow indicate that the trail reenters the state forest slightly ahead on the right.

The trail begins climbing immediately and rises 100 feet over the next 0.25 mile. Pass an old forest road near the apex of this climb and then intersect the gravel Cortland Three Road at 3.25 miles overall. Continue straight across the road, following the orange paints. About 0.3 mile farther when you reach a Y, bear right and continue to follow orange paints along this wide logging road. The trail begins a long descent of 400 feet over the next 0.75 mile. Just after a sign reading "Steep Hill," the road intersects the FLT; turn right and head north along the FLT.

The trail weaves along the contours of the hill through a mixture of pines and hardwoods and is mostly level until you cross a stream 0.5 mile ahead. The stream lies slightly downhill from the parking area at the corner of Odell and Baldwin Roads. After scrambling up the incline, you will emerge just south of this parking area, for a total trip length of 4.8 miles.

Directions

From I-81, take Exit 11/NY 13 toward Cortland/Ithaca. Note that you are following NY 13 through Cortland even though it joins several roads. Follow NY 13 South/Clinton Avenue southeast for 0.2 mile and turn left to stay on NY 13/Church Street. After 0.8 mile, turn right to stay on NY 13/Port Watson Street, and then continue straight at the light, at 0.1 mile, following NY 13/Tompkins Street. After 0.3 mile, turn left on NY 215 South/Owego Street. After 6.1 miles, reach the town of Virgil and turn left onto NY 392 East. Take the first right onto Van Donsel Road, at 0.2 mile. Follow it for 1.6 miles, and turn left on Odell Road. The parking area is 0.8 mile ahead at the junction with Baldwin Road.

Finger Lakes National Forest: Burnt Hill Trail

SCENERY: ★ ★ ★
TRAIL CONDITION: ★ ★ ★ ★
CHILDREN: ★ ★ ★
DIFFICULTY: ★ ★ ★
SOLITUDE: ★ ★ ★ ★ ★

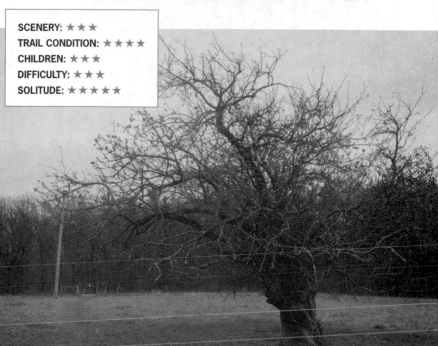

GPS TRAILHEAD COORDINATES: N42° 27.304' W76° 47.180'

DISTANCE & CONFIGURATION: 7.8-mile loop

HIKING TIME: 2.5–3.5 hours

HIGHLIGHTS: Quiet woodland, ponds, open fields, isolated glens

ELEVATION: 1,345' at lower trailhead; 1,842' at highest point along trail

ACCESS: Open 24/7; no fees or permits required

MAPS: Finger Lakes Trail Conference Interloken Trail: Sheet I1; Finger Lakes National Forest map: **www.fs.usda.gov/main/fingerlakes/maps-pubs**; also sometimes available at kiosks

FACILITIES: None

WHEELCHAIR ACCESS: No

COMMENTS: Sections of the trail pass through pasturelands that are actively used May 15–October 31. Cattle gates are employed to keep livestock in, so take care to close gates after passing through. Sections of the trail are shared with equestrians and mountain bikers.

CONTACTS: Finger Lakes National Forest, Hector Ranger District, 607-546-4470, **www.fs.usda.gov/fingerlakes**

Finger Lakes National Forest: Burnt Hill Trail

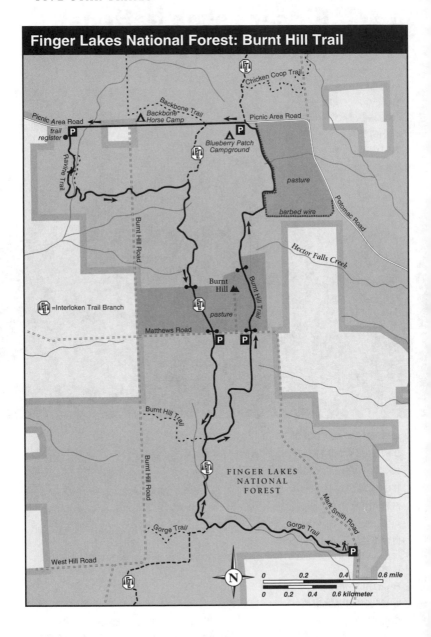

Overview

Unique to the area and to New York, the trails at Finger Lakes National Forest are the only hiking trails within the state that reside on federal land. There are no national parks in New York—only national monuments, heritage areas, memorials, and this one national forest. Also unusual for the trails featured in this book is the combination of woodland and pastureland, which breaks up the typical woodland stroll and provides views of the surrounding landscape.

Route Details

A dark brown sign with white lettering, on the north end of the parking area along Mark Smith Road, indicates that the Gorge and Interloken Trails are on the opposite side of the road and marked with dark blue paints. Follow the dark blue paints southwest up a small hill. Just as a gully comes into sight on the left, the trail swings right and follows this "gorge" westward. First weaving along the gully's slopes and then briefly within, the Gorge Trail ends at a little over 0.75 mile, where it intersects the Interloken Trail. At the intersection, trail signs indicate the distance covered as 1 mile, but my GPS and map software agree that it's just over 0.75 mile.

Bear right and follow the Interloken Trail (marked in orange) northward 0.5 mile to the intersection with the Burnt Hill Trail. The

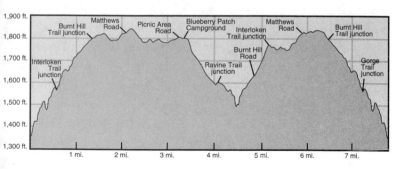

Interloken Trail continues straight ahead; this is the point to which you return when you complete the loop. The Burnt Hill Trail, marked in very faded blue paints, runs both to the east and west. The path west, to your left, leads 0.25 mile to Burnt Hill Road. To follow the loop, turn right and follow the forest road eastward briefly before turning sharply left and heading almost due north. The road continues north 0.25 mile, swings briefly eastward, and then swings north again and reaches Matthews Road at just shy of 2 miles overall. Two alternative parking areas are located along this road and are commonly used by people looking for direct access to the pastureland just ahead.

Based on the moniker *national forest,* you might be surprised to learn that 4,500 of the 16,212 total acres are open pasture. Ranchers use the federal lands for forage for approximately 1,500 head of cattle May 15–October 31. Though forage on public lands is common practice out west, this particular multiuse approach to administering public lands in New York is uncommon. Eighty miles of fencing enclose these pastures, so you have to pass through a narrow cattle gate to continue the trail.

Out in the open pasture, there are no trail signs to guide you, but a worn rut in the grass marks the way through to the pasture exit gate about 0.4 mile to the north. The trail reenters the forest and continues north about 0.25 mile, where it takes a sharp right. In another 0.25 mile, it takes a sharp left just as the trail leads up to another open field. The trail follows this pasture and its barbed wire fence north, then east, and then north again. There are no trail markers along this section, but it's easy to follow the worn path beside the fence. The trail eventually reaches Picnic Area Road and another parking area at just shy of 3.2 miles overall. Across the road is the continuation of the Interloken Trail as well as the Potomac Trails. However, the Burnt Hill loop described follows Picnic Area Road 0.9 mile due west to the beginning of the Ravine Trail.

A short way along Picnic Area Road, you pass the Blueberry Patch Campground entrance on the left (see description of camping in "Nearby Attractions" on page 156). Past the campground is the intersection with the Backbone Trail across the road to the right and the Interloken Trail on the left. If you wish to shorten the loop by about 1.5 miles, turn left here and follow the Interloken Trail 0.3 mile to the intersection with Ravine Trail. For the longer and more scenic route, continue west along Picnic Area Road past the intersection with Burnt Hill Road, and look for the Ravine Trail signs on your left, at 4.1 miles overall.

Shortly after starting the Ravine Trail, you pass a trail register, followed by a fork. The Ravine Trail could be hiked as a stand-alone 1.5-mile loop, and this would be the return point. For the more scenic route back to the Interloken Trail, turn right at the fork and follow the blue paints. The trail follows a stream on the left that has cut a steeply sided hemlock-lined ravine. At first the trail is high above the scenic gorge but eventually winds down to the streambed at about 0.25 mile from the loop sign. Just ahead, you reach the back of the loop and intersect a crossover trail, marked in blue, that leads back to Burnt Hill Road and then onward to the Interloken Trail. The loop trail, also marked in blue, is on the left and leads back to the Picnic Area Road parking area. Bear right to climb out of the ravine and reach Burnt Hill Road in about 0.25 mile. Bear right as you cross the road and continue climbing another 150 feet over the next 0.3 mile to where the trail re-intersects with the Interloken Trail, marked in orange. Turn right and soon cross the first of several planked boardwalks along the trek south back to the first pasture you crossed earlier, 0.5 mile ahead.

Pass through a cattle gate and begin a 0.25-mile slow climb southward across the pasture. Don't forget to look out to your right and backward to take in the broad vista opening across the western horizon. The end of the pasture and exit gate are just past a solitary apple tree near Matthews Road. Across the road is another small parking area and the trail re-intersects the Burnt Hill Trail 0.5 mile ahead. This concludes the loop, and from here you'll return 0.5 mile south via the Interloken Trail to the Gorge Trail and follow it 0.75

mile west, back to the parking area along Mark Smith Road, for a total trip length of 7.8 miles.

Nearby Attractions

I first visited the Finger Lakes National Forest when I coauthored *Best Tent Camping: New York State,* and I considered including the campgrounds in that book. Isolated and not well known, it seemed a good choice. The reason it was not included was that, of the many camping opportunities available on the federal lands, only nine are for car campers, all within the Blueberry Patch Campground. Camping at Potomac Campground is for groups of 10–40, while camping at Backbone Campground is for equestrians. Should you choose to camp at Blueberry Patch, note that facilities are limited to vault toilets and, as is the case elsewhere, there are no water sources in any campgrounds. Backpackers, however, will find a multitude of opportunities for camping in the backcountry. The main regulation to be aware of is that you must camp farther than 50 feet from streams, ponds, developed areas, and trails. In addition, camping in the pastures is prohibited May 15–October 31. Camping at trail shelters is limited to two nights.

Directions

From Watkins Glen: At the intersection of NY 414 North and NY 79 East just north of Watkins Glen, bear right onto NY 79 East. Follow it 1.6 miles, and turn right to continue along NY 79 East. At 3.8 miles, turn left onto Mark Smith Road. The parking area is 0.7 mile ahead on the right.

   From Ithaca: Follow NY 79 West out of Ithaca. At 15.3 miles, turn right onto Mark Smith Road. The parking area is 0.7 mile ahead on the right.

20 **Buttermilk Falls State Park: Gorge Trail**

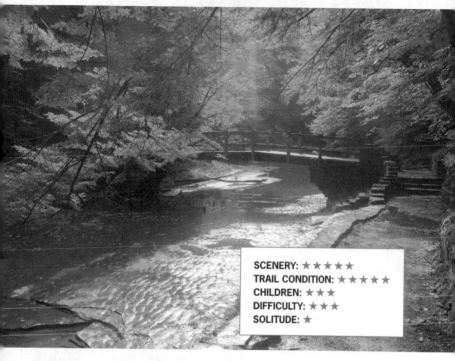

SCENERY: ★ ★ ★ ★ ★
TRAIL CONDITION: ★ ★ ★ ★ ★
CHILDREN: ★ ★ ★
DIFFICULTY: ★ ★ ★
SOLITUDE: ★

GPS TRAILHEAD COORDINATES: N42° 24.976'   W76° 31.285'

DISTANCE & CONFIGURATION: 1.6-mile loop (See Lake Treman Loop, page 164, for an extended trip.)

HIKING TIME: 1–1.5 hours

HIGHLIGHTS: Waterfalls, scenic gorge

ELEVATION: 420' at trailhead; 870' at top of gorge

ACCESS: Daily, sunrise–sunset; Gorge Trail open only spring–early November; $7 vehicle entrance fee

MAPS: nysparks.com/parks/151/maps.aspx; also available at entrance booth

FACILITIES: Restrooms, concessions, swimming area, picnic area, campground

WHEELCHAIR ACCESS: Yes, but in day-use area only, not along trail

COMMENTS: The Gorge Trail opens in the spring, but only after safety inspections and required repairs are complete. Check with the park if you plan to visit in early spring.

CONTACTS: Buttermilk Falls State Park, 607-273-5761, **nysparks.com/parks/151/details.aspx**

Buttermilk Falls State Park: Gorge Trail

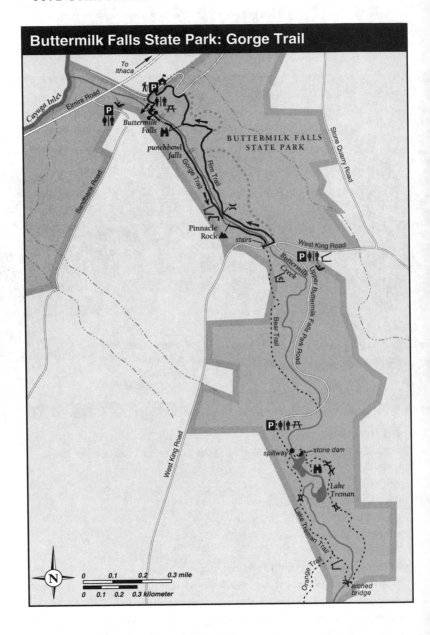

To Ithaca

Cayuga Inlet

Elmira Road

Buttermilk Falls

punchbowl falls

Sandbank Road

Gorge Trail

Rim Trail

BUTTERMILK FALLS STATE PARK

Stone Quarry Road

Pinnacle Rock

stairs

West King Road

Buttermilk Creek

Upper Buttermilk Falls Park Road

Bear Trail

West King Road

spillway

stone dam

Lake Treman

Lake Treman Trail

Orange Trail

arched bridge

N

| 0 | 0.1 | 0.2 | 0.3 mile |
| 0 | 0.1 | 0.2 | 0.3 kilometer |

Overview

Waterfalls, dramatic waterscapes, and handsome stonework are all iconic images of the state parks in the Finger Lakes region. The Gorge Trail at Buttermilk Falls won't let you down in providing all these scenic settings in abundance. The plunge pools and potholes are particularly striking, and you'll find plenty of opportunities to snap gorgeous pictures.

Route Details

To reach the Gorge Trail, make your way through the day-use area, over a small bridge crossing Buttermilk Creek, to a paved path and an iron gate. In the summer, the swimming area beneath Buttermilk Falls will attract crowds, while tourists will be plentiful in any season. You might find yourself shoulder to shoulder with photographers and sightseers along the narrow bridge, and people often crowd the initial set of stone steps for additional photo ops. Rest assured that the crowds dissipate quickly as hikers and groups find their own pace and spread out along the trail.

The trail climbs up stone steps to the right of the lower portion of Buttermilk Falls. The falls consists of two sections: the lower falls visible here and an upper falls whose lower section is visible a short distance ahead. Both falls are estimated to be 80–90 feet tall and consist

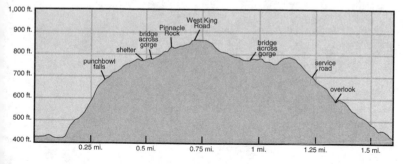

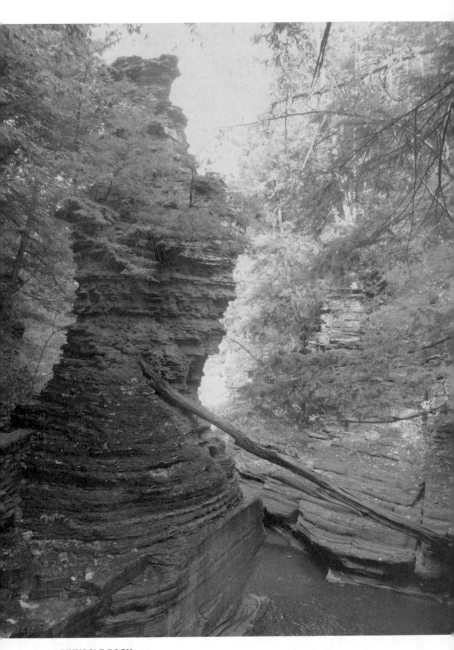

PINNACLE ROCK

mainly of tumbling and frothy slides, whose foamy character likely prompted the falls' moniker. You soon reach the top of the initial climb beside the crest of the lower falls. To your left is a handsome stone lookout. This is a great spot to gaze back down onto the park entrance and day-use area, and also to take in Ithaca farther to the north. Turn south and you will be able to see the bottom of the upper falls.

Back along the trail, continue up the stairs to your right, travel up a switchback, and emerge near a fenced-in area beside the gorge. The chain-link fence on your left shields you from the sheer cliffs that encompass the upper section of the falls. A little farther ahead you glimpse where the upper section of the gorge spills into the lower section that encompassed Buttermilk Falls. Sometimes referred to as a punch bowl falls, the water shoots out of a square cut in the gorge walls and drops into the sheer-walled basin. Unfortunately, surrounding foliage obscures the view, so a late-fall visit might be your best option for taking in this dramatic scene. Obscured or not, the scene is impressive and provides a dramatic introduction to the true gorge ahead.

Proceed up a series of concrete steps at the conclusion of which most of the steep climbing is finished. Although the trail continues to ascend the next 0.5 mile, the grade is gentler, and short sections of stone stairs aid in your ascent. After passing the punch bowl falls, which are approximately 25 feet tall, the gorge narrows and you will travel much of the time within the gorge itself, often within feet of the water. Weaving your way beside sheer cliffs on your right, with equally imposing escarpments and dramatic waterscapes to your left, provides a feature-rich trip and a shutterbug's delight. This is typical of many of the Finger Lakes gorges, but, though many have similar features, each possesses its own unique character. A case in point is the stunning example of potholes along Buttermilk Creek. Practically circular in shape, the potholes were formed originally as plunge pools at the bases of previous waterfalls. As the tops of these falls eroded away, the undercut portion of the stream remained and trapped rocks and sediment inside. These sediments and rocks cycle about inside each hole in a whirlpool-like motion, further widening and deepening the pothole. As you enter the gorge, you will see the first of many of these striking potholes.

You will pass by additional potholes, as well as multiple small falls or flumes with their related plunge pools in quick succession, each picturesque and fascinating. Soon the chain-link fence ends, and the gorge practically engulfs you. Stone walkways and short stone walls line the path in a harmonious and aesthetically pleasing way that makes the chain-link fence seem almost an affront. As you wind up a series of stone steps, lined with mossy stone walls, beside a short waterfall, you will know what I mean. The hardscape and landscape intertwine onward all along the trail, and rather than describe each, I'll let the features surprise and intrigue you in turn.

A little under 0.5 mile along, pass by a small fork in the trail that leads up to the right, where a wooden trail shelter sits above the trail. The main trail continues on your left, goes down a set of stairs, passes a small bench set into the rock wall beside the trail, and then comes out onto a relatively flat walkway where a wooden bridge spans Buttermilk Creek. The bridge leads to a small spur trail that connects with the Rim Trail. You could use this spur to return, but you would be missing the next big feature along the trail.

Straight ahead the trail curves eastward under a steep cliff as it follows a slight bend in Buttermilk Creek. Before you is a long staircase on the right, with a series of square and shallow falls to the left. This scene is picturesque all on its own, but as you climb nearer to the top of these falls and round the corner, Pinnacle Rock comes into view. Reminiscent of some type of organic castle tower, Pinnacle Rock is a tall spire that looms 40 feet above the trail. Make your way through a narrow passage at its base, and you'll notice a deep, almost green, pothole that adds to the spire's peculiarity.

Continuing forward, the gorge's sheer walls diminish, but the striking waterscapes do not. Tiny falls, flumes, plunge pools, and potholes riddle the creek, and you can almost imagine that this is how the gorge looked when it began to form thousands of years ago. The Gorge Trail continues less than 0.25 mile with the grade leveling off, and you soon reach a bridge along West King Road. Stairs lead up to the road where the upper portion of the park begins. At this point you have a choice: Continue across the road and onto the Bear Trail to make a circuit around Lake Treman for a round-trip of 4.8 miles, or return to the lower parking area. I highly recommend the added circuit around Lake Treman (described on the following pages), where a woodland stroll followed by a shallow lake and intricate stonework await. If you choose to end your hike, you have a choice of returning along the Rim Trail (to your left and across the bridge) or returning the way you came, which I strongly advise. However, if you're like me and a stickler for hiking loop trails to avoid retracing your steps whenever possible, then you will return along the Rim Trail.

The Rim Trail is pretty uneventful and lacks much in scenery, but I will outline some of the mileage markers. A quarter mile along the Rim Trail (1 mile overall), reach an intersection with a spur trail down to a bridge. Shortly after, when you intersect a service road, follow that service road briefly before bearing left back onto the foot trail. At 0.6 mile (1.4 miles overall), pass a lookout on the left that is across from the stone lookout along the Gorge Trail. The lower parking area is approximately 0.25 mile farther, for a round-trip of 1.6 miles, or 4.8 miles if you include the Lake Treman Loop.

Directions

From the intersection of NY 79 and NY 13/NY 34 in Ithaca, continue south along NY 13/NY 34/NY 96/Elmira Road. Turn left onto Buttermilk Falls Road, 1.1 miles. Parking is just past the entrance gate.

21 Buttermilk Falls State Park: Lake Treman Loop

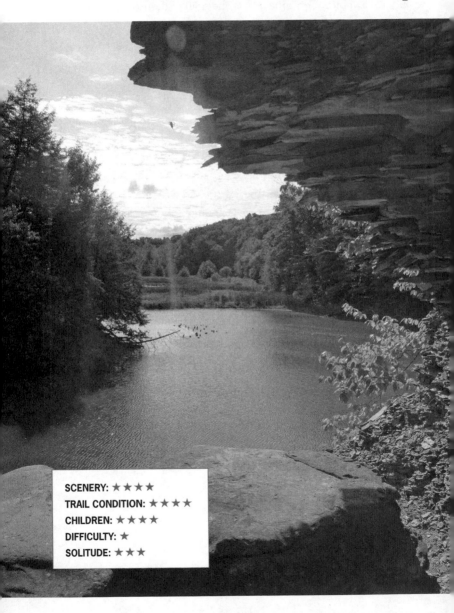

SCENERY: ★ ★ ★ ★
TRAIL CONDITION: ★ ★ ★ ★
CHILDREN: ★ ★ ★ ★
DIFFICULTY: ★
SOLITUDE: ★ ★ ★

GPS TRAILHEAD COORDINATES: N42° 24.606'   W76° 30.857'

DISTANCE & CONFIGURATION: 3.2-mile loop from West King Road; 4.8-mile figure eight when combined with Gorge Trail

HIKING TIME: 1–1.5 hours for loop; 2–3 hours total trip time when including the Gorge Trail (see page 157)

HIGHLIGHTS: Shallow lake, wildlife viewing, stone dam

ELEVATION: 870' at trailhead; 1,015' highest point along loop

ACCESS: Daily, sunrise–sunset; sections along and near the dam are closed in winter; $7 vehicle entrance fee

MAPS: nysparks.com/parks/151/maps.aspx; also available at entrance booth

FACILITIES: Restrooms, drinking fountains, picnic areas

WHEELCHAIR ACCESS: No

COMMENTS: The northeast corner of the Lake Treman Loop (the section near and around the dam) is often closed during the winter, while the other sections are typically open year-round. Call ahead or visit the park's website for the most up-to-date trail info.

CONTACTS: Buttermilk Falls State Park, 607-273-5761, **nysparks.com/parks/151 /details.aspx**

Overview

After exploring the turbulent gorge along Buttermilk Creek, Lake Treman is a strikingly calm and placid setting. Wildlife frequents the lake, providing an excellent opportunity for birding and animal observations. Additionally, many visitors who hike the Gorge Trail often eschew the lake loop, allowing for some solitude along the trail as well. While much of the trail consists of worn footpaths, the stone dam found on the north end of the lake is another example of harmoniously constructed stonework built into the landscape.

Route Details

Most hikers will be adding this trail as an extension of the Gorge Trail, which I highly recommend (see Gorge Trail, page 157). For those visitors choosing to explore only Lake Treman, you have two options. You may park at the parking area located just past the upper vehicle entrance and follow the Bear Trail as described here. Or you could take the park road farther south to another parking area just

Buttermilk Falls State Park: Lake Treman Loop

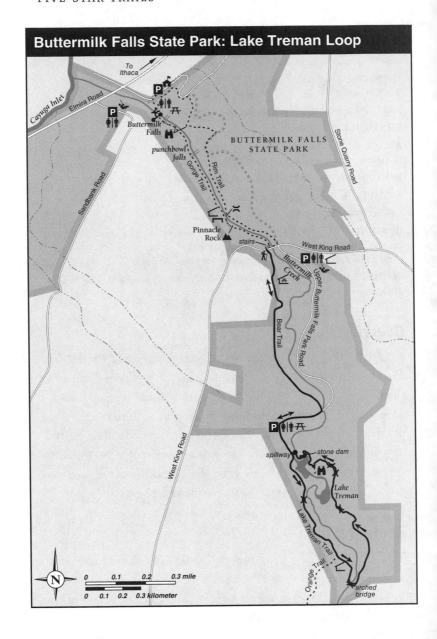

before the lake loop trailhead. For simplicity's sake, the trail detailed below, including mileage, begins at the end of the Gorge Trail where it intersects West King Road.

The initial leg of this trip is along the Bear Trail, 0.75 mile long, and is a mostly level footpath that weaves through the hardwood forest that surrounds Buttermilk Creek. The creek takes on an entirely new character after the dramatic gorge behind you. Mostly flat and meandering, the creek is more like a delta, with broad, flat sections beside the creek that act as a floodplain when the creek is full during high water. This is a favorite habitat for sycamore trees, whose odd mottled and peeling bark always stands out in northeastern forests. An impressive stand of these trees is located approximately midway along this leg to the trail. You'll make quick time along this section of trail and reach its end near a small waterfall. The trail opens out onto a broad mowed lawn that flanks the park road. Bear right along this road and follow it less than 0.25 mile to a picnic area and parking lot. The picnic area, to your left, sits below a waterfall along Lake Treman's spillway. During dry times, as when I visited, the falls are on the quiet side, but they make excellent company should you decide to take a break here before proceeding along the lake loop.

Head past the restrooms on your right and up a gravel drive to the northern tip of Lake Treman, where you reach the top of the spillway. A short wooden bridge crosses the square-cut channel on your

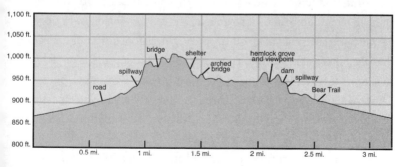

left, and this is where you will be returning when you complete the lake circuit. For now, bear right to make a counterclockwise circuit of the lake. The gravel footpath, marked with white paints, climbs slightly until you are well above the lake with some interesting views of a cliff-lined cove along the lake to the northeast. You can't quite make it out to the dam there.

The dam was built in the fall of 1930 to help control the flow of Buttermilk Creek through the park. Lake Treman was created as a result, and looking out on the lake you'll notice that it is not very deep. The lake is more akin to a shallow depression than the deeply cut bodies of water found elsewhere in the region. Riddled with many cattails and gravel bars, the lake has an ideal habitat for wildlife, which you're likely to view. At 1.1 miles, you'll cross a short wooden bridge and shortly after weave your way down closer to the lake. Not far ahead, you reach an intersection with an orange-marked trail. This spur trail is part of the Finger Lakes Trail and leads to Sweedler Preserve at Lick Brook (described on page 182). Continue straight, south, past a trail shelter on your left, and you will soon come to a broad, open area beside the headwaters of the lake. Continue along the gravel bar to a handsome arched bridge that crosses Buttermilk Creek, roughly 0.5 mile along the lake loop and the midpoint of the trip. On the other side you will follow a broad forest road on your way back north.

The road comes to an end about 0.25 mile ahead, as you turn to your right and climb up concrete steps. The trail briefly follows a ridge between the lake and valley off to your right, before descending near the lake. There are multiple spots to look out along the lake along this leg of the trip, but some of the most interesting vantage points lie farther ahead. After passing through a few wet areas, you'll pass a small hemlock grove on your left. The heavily shaded hilltop sits high above the lake and provides multiple places to look south on the lake but also glimpse the cliff-lined cove and stone dam to the north. Lots of interesting photos can be taken here or at a couple more lookouts farther along the trail.

At a little over 2 miles, the trail switches back southward and descends along stone steps cut into the surrounding cliffs to the top of the dam. The dam top, mere feet above the lake to your left and 36 feet down to the creek bottom on your right, is only several feet across. Steel posts with wire rails guard the sheer drop-off, but those with an aversion to heights might want to keep to the lake side of the path. Again, you can't help but marvel at the intricate stonework here. The dam and even the staircases that lead to and from its top seem to grow out of the landscape.

Once across the dam, a curved staircase brings you over a small shale hill, and you will soon find yourself back at the wooden bridge over the lake spillway. From here it is another mile back the way you came to West King Road or 1.8 miles back to the parking area at the lower entrance to the Gorge Trail.

Directions

For those combining this trip with the Gorge Trail, see the directions for Buttermilk Falls: Gorge Trail on page 163. For direct access to the Lake Treman Loop, follow the directions for Buttermilk Falls, but continue 0.1 mile farther south along NY 13/NY 34/NY 96/Elmira Road. Turn left on West King Road, and follow it 1.2 miles to the upper park entrance on your right.

Texas Hollow State Forest

22

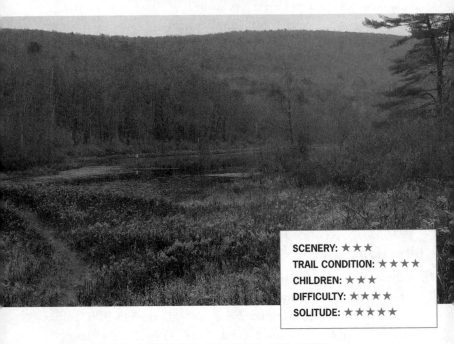

SCENERY: ★ ★ ★
TRAIL CONDITION: ★ ★ ★ ★
CHILDREN: ★ ★ ★
DIFFICULTY: ★ ★ ★ ★
SOLITUDE: ★ ★ ★ ★ ★

GPS TRAILHEAD COORDINATES: N42° 24.751'   W76° 47.531'

DISTANCE & CONFIGURATION: 2.6-mile out-and-back; 4.8 miles total (including alternate routes)

HIKING TIME: 2–3 hours

HIGHLIGHTS: Quiet woodland, ponds, wetlands

ELEVATION: 1,215' at lower trailhead; 1,770' at upper trailhead

ACCESS: Open 24/7; no fees or permits required

MAPS: Finger Lakes Trail Conference: Sheet M15; DEC Texas Hollow map: **dec.ny.gov /lands/37445.html**

FACILITIES: None

WHEELCHAIR ACCESS: No

COMMENTS: The designated parking area for the trail is along the east side of Texas Hollow Road, along a short access road and just in front of a vehicle barrier gate. Parking is recommended here, as the large gravel road farther north, though intersected by the Finger Lakes Trail, is on private property.

CONTACTS: Division of Lands & Forests, DEC Bath Sub-Office, 607-776-2165, **dec.ny.gov/lands/37445.html**

Overview

Within the 937-acre Texas Hollow State Forest is a large man-made pond as well as several natural ponds and bogs. The setting is ideal for wildlife, and this seldom-traveled path provides lots of solitude in which to immerse yourself. A long 600-foot climb offers a welcome challenge for hikers seeking a bit more difficulty or conditioning.

Route Details

To begin the trail, head south past the vehicle barrier gate and downhill. At the bottom of the hill, pass the intersection with the Finger Lakes Trail (FLT) and continue toward the large pond ahead. The trail continues along the north end of the pond, atop a man-made dike and past an overgrown flood control grate that bubbles loudly on your right. Follow the top of the berm; then proceed up a short hill and reach a trail intersection. On your left is a blue-marked diversion loop, while straight ahead is the return leg of the trip, the white-marked Finger Lakes/North Country Trail. Turn left, and follow the blue paints up over a small hillock into a hemlock grove. Off to your left is a small pond, while a broad wetland is visible to your right. The trail gradually bends its way eastward, and you soon pass an area where beavers have felled numerous saplings. This opening along the trail is roughly 0.5 mile from the start. Just past this clearing, you have panoramic views across the marsh. Notice how the opposing Foots Hill is shaped: long with a flat top and steep 500-foot-high sides. These are the common characteristics of the oversteepened hills in the region. Once V-shaped, these river/stream tributary valleys were bulldozed by Pleistocene-era glaciers into broad U-shaped valleys whose drainage is far smaller than the eroded hillsides would suggest.

Continue past this opening up a hill into more hemlocks. A short distance later, the trail briefly joins an old forest road that comes in from the left and continues southward as it makes a circuit around the wetland. Shy of a mile, it reconnects with the Finger Lakes Trail. To your right is the return to the parking area, while

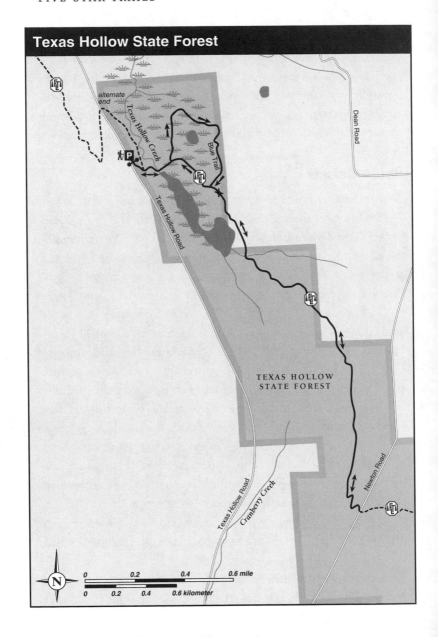

Texas Hollow State Forest

to the left is our route farther into Texas Hollow. Continue east, to your left, and pass over a couple of short 2-foot-wide bridges that cross small wet areas in quick succession. Along this route you will no doubt have seen another wet area sprawling off on your right; this is the backwater behind the dam along Texas Hollow Creek. As the trail approaches the open water, you reach one of the sections of private property that the trail crosses through. Much of the Finger Lakes Trail system passes through private property and, for the sake of this continued cooperation, please remain on the trail.

After a little less than 1.25 miles, you cross a seasonal stream. At the time I visited in fall, the stream had run dry, but its course was obvious by the washed-out sections of shale and cut banks. What was not immediately evident at the time was the spot where the trail continued on the opposing bank. Fallen leaves obscured the worn path, and the trail's white paint tends to blend in with the trees' lightly colored bark. Most trails are well marked even though the blazes are sometimes hard to see, but should you ever lose the path, simply look back on the blazes behind you and you'll be able to predict the general direction the trail may follow. Furthermore, double paints indicate a change in direction along the trail, so be mindful if you see those behind you. I have no doubt that the trail is more discernible in the summer, but just in case look slightly to your left, and the paints/path should come into view.

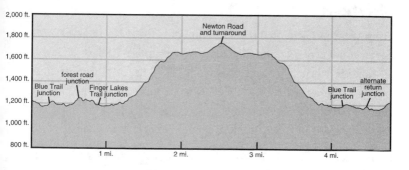

Up until this point, the trail has stayed mostly flat, but the path forward involves a bit of climbing—600 feet of elevation gain over the next 1.25 miles. The steepest sections are near the beginning of the climb, and though it levels off near the end, it is still ascending. Along this climb you will intersect and cross two logging roads and then intersect and follow a third forest road southward. The grade eases a bit along this portion, and roughly 0.5 mile from the end of the climb, you'll pass through the remnants of a boundary stone wall with cobbles strewn to both sides of the trail. As you near the end of the trip, you pass through a series of small switchbacks and come out on Newtown Road. You have covered roughly 2.6 miles so far. Return the way you came, but to add just a touch of diversity along the trail, I suggest that you forgo the blue bypass and continue straight along the Finger Lakes Trail once you return to that intersection.

If you wish to extend your hike a little farther, just shy of 0.5 mile, you can again continue along the Finger Lakes Trail, this time at the intersection just past the pond and below the path up to the vehicle barrier gate. Instead of returning to your car at the gate, follow the white paints and Texas Hollow Creek roughly 0.3 mile northward. The trail is mostly flat until the very end, where it climbs up quickly to intersect Texas Hollow Road again. Turn left and follow Texas Hollow Road back to your car.

Directions

From Watkins Glen: At the intersection of NY 414 North and NY 79 East just north of Watkins Glen, bear right onto NY 79 East. Follow it 1.6 miles and turn right to continue along NY 79 East. At 2.3 miles, turn right onto Texas Hollow Road. Follow it 1.2 miles south. The parking area is in front of a vehicle barrier gate on the left side of the road, less than 0.25 mile past where the FLT crosses Texas Hollow Road.

From Ithaca: Follow NY 79 West out of Ithaca. At 14.8 miles, turn left to stay on NY 79 West. Turn left onto Texas Hollow Road at 2 miles, and follow directions above.

23 Robert H. Treman State Park: Enfield Glen

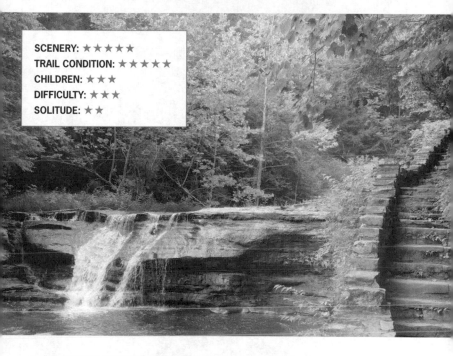

SCENERY: ★ ★ ★ ★ ★
TRAIL CONDITION: ★ ★ ★ ★ ★
CHILDREN: ★ ★ ★
DIFFICULTY: ★ ★ ★
SOLITUDE: ★ ★

GPS TRAILHEAD COORDINATES: N42° 23.890'   W76° 33.427'

DISTANCE & CONFIGURATION: 4.5-mile loop

HIKING TIME: 2–3 hours

HIGHLIGHTS: Waterfalls, scenic gorge, quiet woodland

ELEVATION: 480' at lower trailhead; 920' at upper parking area

ACCESS: Daily, sunrise–sunset; Enfield Glen Gorge Trail open only spring–early November; $7 vehicle entrance fee

MAPS: nysparks.com/parks/135/maps.aspx; also available at park office

FACILITIES: Restrooms, concessions, swimming area, picnic area, campground

WHEELCHAIR ACCESS: Yes, along a short trail to the swimming area and lower falls, but not along trail described here

COMMENTS: The Enfield Glen Gorge Trail opens in the spring, but only after safety inspections and required repairs are complete. Check with the park if you plan to visit in early spring.

CONTACTS: Robert H. Treman State Park, 607-273-3440, **nysparks.com/parks/135 /details.aspx**

Robert H. Treman State Park: Enfield Glen

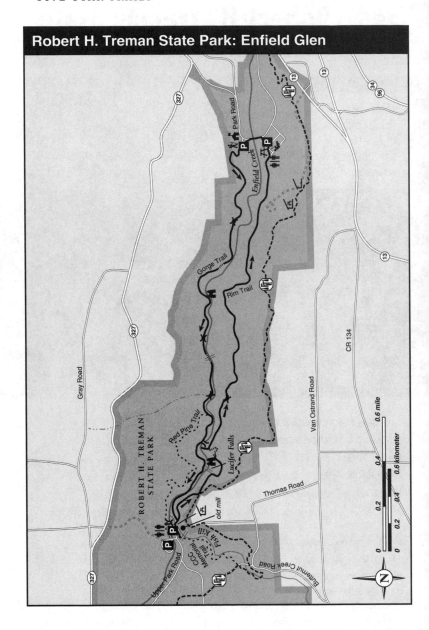

Overview

Also known as Enfield Glen, the Gorge Trail at Robert H. Treman State Park is yet another example of the beautiful waterfalls and gorges that surround Ithaca. Unlike other gorge trails, whose features welcome you from the start, the waterscapes at Enfield Glen begin small and placid and grow ever wilder and stunning as the trail progresses. The drama peaks with the towering 115-foot Lucifer Falls.

Route Details

Trails through scenic gorges seem to be around every corner in the Ithaca area. But don't let their frequency beguile you into thinking they are all the same. True, many are part of the state park system and, as such, share common characteristics like swimming areas, campgrounds, picnic facilities, and a general level of development along the trails (such as stone staircases or hardened paths). However, the natural features these trails encompass set each one apart and create very different settings. Watkins Glen is a marvel of stonework and narrow passages, Buttermilk Falls has plunge pools and stark potholes, Taughannock Falls is less a gorge and more a canyon, and here, at Robert H. Treman State Park, Lucifer Falls reigns supreme.

The Gorge Trail begins along a paved walkway, to the left of the park office, followed by a steep climb through a hemlock forest.

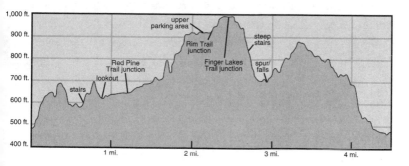

Over the next 0.25 mile the trail gains 200 feet in elevation but, after this initial climb, remains mostly flat with only modest descents and climbs until you begin to ascend out of the lower gorge and approach the crest of Lucifer Falls, more than 1.5 miles farther along. Unlike at other gorge trails, the dramatic waterscapes are slow to reveal themselves here. Indeed the first waterfall within the park, the 70-foot-high Lower Falls that feeds the swimming area, can be heard only along the initial section of the Gorge Trail. You first encounter Enfield Creek near a small flume, but the sojourn along the creek is brief, and soon after the trail climbs away from the creek up a long set of stairs and back into the forest. Just under 1 mile in, you hike along a small narrow ridge with a chain-link fence to either side. At the conclusion of this narrow corridor, you reach a small stone lookout above a small waterfall. From the lookout, the trail turns sharply right and down a set of stairs to the creek bed again. The trail remains in the gorge and beside the creek from this point forward, though now the gorge feels more like a floodplain than a chasm. Shortly after crossing a wooden bridge, you spot a waterfall ahead. At 10 feet tall, this serene little waterfall cascades to the left of a handsome set of stone stairs. You are now approximately 1.25 miles from the trailhead.

Less than 0.25 mile farther, you reach a wooden bridge that crosses a small feeder stream and make a short descent to a deep and broad pool. Looming ahead is a steep shale wall that towers over the trail on the right side. The trail curves around the base of this cliff and soon passes by the intersection with the Red Pine Trail on your right. Just past this intersection, you come upon another small waterfall along Enfield Creek. Worn footpaths lead down to the creek bed, where you can get some decent photos of the square waterfall; however, the view is slightly obstructed. Don't worry; farther along the trail are better viewing points from above, or if you want a panoramic shot of the base, a vantage point across the creek is easily accessible along the return leg of the trip.

Follow the trail to the right and above the falls, where shortly after you encounter another tiny cascade. Ahead is a wooden bridge and steep outcrop that slants above the trail. The bridge leads across Enfield Creek and connects to the lower portion of the Rim Trail, but our destination is straight ahead. The trail begins a steep ascent, first up some steps followed by a broad stone path. As you round a corner along the trail, you'll notice that the trail fence becomes more substantial, first log and rail, then log and stone pillar, and finally solid stone walls. Once around the corner, you catch your first view of the 115-foot Lucifer Falls. The basin surrounding the falls is hundreds of feet high, and the verdant cliff face opposing the falls provides an interesting contrast. No doubt you will find yourself snapping multiple panoramic photos. It should be noted that the view of Lucifer Falls is from the side, but along the return leg of the trip, you have the opportunity to view it head-on from a lookout. More than likely, you will be able to spot that lookout from here. Try to picture yourself there, and I have no doubt that you will be surprised at what you see once you are there and looking back down.

The stonework that makes the paths, walls, and staircases is substantial, some of it the remnants of Civilian Conservation Corps (CCC) work from the 1930s (see the Watkins Glen trail description, page 194, for more about the CCC's work in the area). A particularly handsome example of the work done here is the arched staircase that leads to the top of the falls. Once up the stairs, the trail turns to the right and follows Enfield Creek in a square-cut channel atop the falls. Even more intricate stonework lines the path here, as you weave your way past a short cascade and then through the now narrow gorge. Soon an arched stone bridge carries you over the creek, where some interesting cataracts and flumes create another picturesque setting. Again the contrast between nature's stone carving and human craft provides an interesting juxtaposition. You'll pass a shallow bench cut into the cliff on your left just before passing the last of the falls along this section of the gorge. As soon as you pass these falls you are thrust out into the upper park, a change that is actually a bit jarring. The open fields and bustle of activity around the parking area and upper visitor center seems all too sudden after you've so recently been hemmed in by cliffs in the middle of a rugged gorge.

To continue the loop, head toward the large visitor center at the old mill. If you are in need of refreshment or relief, now is the time to seek it, before beginning the 2.25-mile trek back to the lower parking area. Even if you are itching to get away from the crowds here, it might be worth the short stop by the visitor center, where another waterfall is visible. Certainly no Lucifer Falls, it is a handsome cascade whose force was once harnessed to power a mill here, details of which are inside.

The Rim Trail back begins just past a wooden trail map suspended between two round posts. Head uphill and immediately cross a pair of wooden bridges. You may have noticed blue blazes along the Rim Trail; these blazes are related to the Finger Lakes/North Country Trail. The blue blazes diverge off to your right 0.25 mile along, but we continue along the unblazed trail straight ahead. A little farther along you pass a worn path on your left, while a stone staircase lies ahead. The short path to the left leads to a small lookout where you can view the stairs leading up to Lucifer Falls. The main lookout on the falls is less than 0.25 mile ahead, where a stone wall protects hikers from getting too close to the cliff edge. At the lookout, a stunning panorama of both Lucifer Falls and the stone staircases and walls opens out before you. If you were not impressed with the work before, you cannot help but be amazed now. From this vantage point you really can appreciate how sheer the cliffs are and how tightly the path, previously tread, hugs its contours. In my experience, it was hard to really take in the entire scale of it, but now looking down you have a much deeper understanding.

Continue along the trail a short ways to the long and steep staircase that brings you back to the base of the gorge. Made entirely of stone, the stairs are very steep and switch back on themselves a couple of times. Along the descent you'll have some interesting views of the wooded glen ahead, but also keep an eye out for a small alcove. In this alcove is a memorial plaque to Robert and Laura Treman,

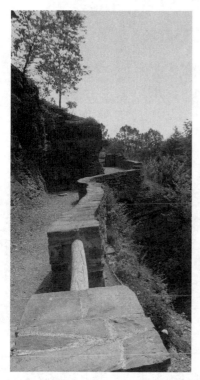

LOOKING BACK AT TRAIL NEAR LUCIFER FALLS

who, as the plaque states, gifted Enfield Glen to the state for all to enjoy. Shortly after passing the alcove, the stairs end and you are back at the bottom of the gorge. A short way ahead is a trail intersection, roughly 2.75 miles from the beginning of your hike. Ahead is the bridge across Enfield Creek that leads to the Gorge Trail, while to the right is the Rim Trail and the return leg of the route described. Head east along the Rim Trail. About 0.25 mile past this intersection, you will pass a footpath to your left. This footpath leads to the square falls previously mentioned. From this side of the creek you have an unobstructed view of the falls and yet another great photo opportunity. From this point forward the trail is a pleasant stroll through the surrounding forest for approximately 1.5 miles back to the trailhead and lower parking area.

Directions

From the intersection of NY 79 and NY 13/NY 34 in Ithaca, continue south along NY 13/NY 34/NY 96/Elmira Road. Turn right on NY 327/Enfield Falls Road, at 2.6 miles (1.5 miles past the entrance to Buttermilk Falls State Park). Take the first left onto Park Road and pay the fee at the entrance gate. Continue 0.7 mile along Park Road to the large parking area near the park office.

24 # Sweedler Preserve
at Lick Brook

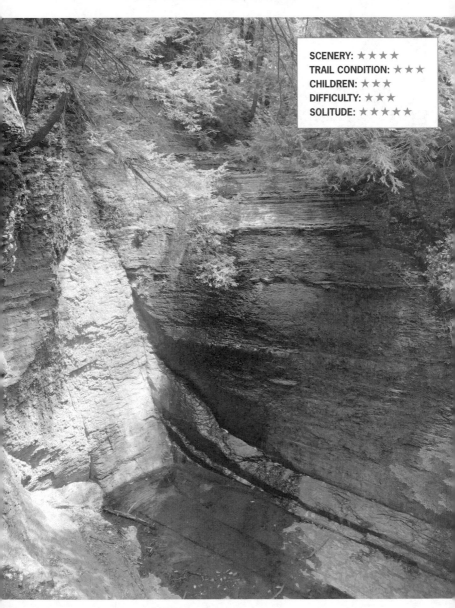

SCENERY: ★ ★ ★ ★
TRAIL CONDITION: ★ ★ ★
CHILDREN: ★ ★ ★
DIFFICULTY: ★ ★ ★
SOLITUDE: ★ ★ ★ ★

GPS TRAILHEAD COORDINATES: N42° 23.745'   W76° 31.995'

DISTANCE & CONFIGURATION: 1.6-mile loop; 0.75-mile side trip

HIKING TIME: 1.5 hours

HIGHLIGHTS: Waterfalls, scenic gorge

ELEVATION: 946' at trailhead; 460' at basin

ACCESS: Daily, sunrise–sunset; no fees or permits required

MAPS: fllt.org (search for "Sweedler Preserve")

FACILITIES: None

WHEELCHAIR ACCESS: No

COMMENTS: Parts of the trail traverse the edge of a sheer cliff, so caution is advised. Because cliff edges are often undercut, approach cautiously and never tread where you are uncertain of your footing. During the height of summer and drought conditions, the creek runs dry, so plan your trip accordingly.

CONTACTS: Finger Lakes Land Trust, 607-275-9487, **fllt.org/protected_lands /protected_lands1.php?id=29**

Overview

Ithaca is known for its beautiful gorges. It's practically a slogan. Most of these scenic wonders are located in state parks and are a popular destination for tourists and locals alike. What many don't know is that this area has lots of other wild gorges outside its state parks. Though not as dramatic as their park brethren, they are nonetheless beautiful. Add the chance to enjoy the gorge and waterfalls in relative solitude, and Sweedler Preserve at Lick Brook will likely be high on your list of places to visit while in the area.

Route Details

I visited this scenic trail after hiking the Robert H. Treman gorge (see trail description on page 175). At the height of summer, the Enfield Creek and falls at Robert H. Treman State Park were flowing. Unfortunately, the same was not true for Lick Brook. Near the trailhead, the creek was wet but not really flowing. Farther along, the falls had run dry, but this really didn't detract from the trail's charms. The creek and trail are relatively undeveloped, and the wild nature of the

Sweedler Preserve at Lick Brook

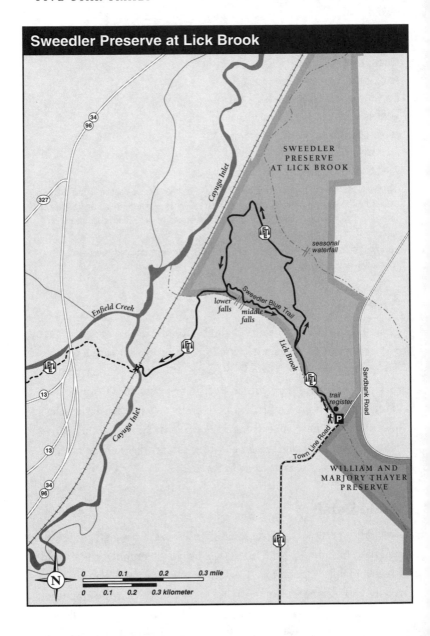

SWEEDLER
PRESERVE
AT LICK BROOK

seasonal
waterfall

Cayuga Inlet

Enfield Creek

Sweedler Blue Trail

lower
falls

middle
falls

Lick Brook

trail
register

Sandbank Road

Cayuga Inlet

Town Line Road

WILLIAM AND
MARJORY THAYER
PRESERVE

N

| 0 | 0.1 | 0.2 | 0.3 mile |
| 0 | 0.1 | 0.2 | 0.3 kilometer |

gorge is enhanced by the fact that you are essentially alone, unlike at nearby state parks.

Parking for the trail is along the west side of Town Line Road. If vehicles are thoughtfully spaced, there is room for approximately 10 cars along the shoulder. The trail is located just before the bridge crossing Lick Brook heading south along Town Line Road. Follow the path northwest 150 feet to the handsome kiosk beside the trail. The kiosk and trail are maintained by the Finger Lakes Land Trust (FLLT) and the Cayuga Trails Club (CTC). I always advise hikers to sign in at trail registers. This is not only safe hiking practice but also incredibly useful for both the state and private trail clubs involved in trail planning and allocation of resources. Continue northwest, past the register, following Lick Brook downstream. Shrouded in thick forest, the creek flows through a channel of eroded limestone with walls that are 10–20 feet high. This shallow gorge has wild nature that only hints at the deeply cut ravine ahead.

As you approach the steep gorge, you will notice property boundary warning signs dotting the opposing bank. The FLLT owns 128 acres on the east side of the creek but not on the opposing bank, so please respect boundaries with private property. Ahead and out of sight the creek disappears into a precipitous ravine, well over 100 feet deep. This is the upper waterfall along Lick Brook and is more than

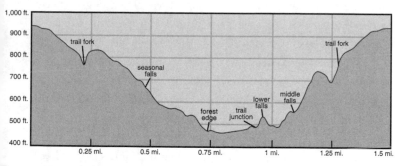

93 feet high and 9 feet wide, but accessing a vantage point to see the actual falls can be difficult and dangerous. Unlike at state parks, no fences or guard rails prevent wayward hikers from the sheer drop, so proceed with caution when inspecting the gorge. Cliffs are often undercut, and soil along these edges can be unstable, so venturing too close to the edge is strongly discouraged. A good rule of thumb when exploring this sort of geography is not to venture too close to an edge you have not observed from another vantage point. If you can't verify that it is safe, don't risk it because there are plenty of beautiful vantage points farther along.

In less than 0.25 mile from the start, you reach a fork in the trail. To the left, marked in blue, is the return trail that hugs the gorge's edge. This approach is steep, and I found that you will have better glimpses of the gorge while climbing than descending. The trail to the right, marked with white paint, winds through the surrounding forest to another lesser gorge and a seasonal waterfall. This white trail makes the 400-foot descent over a 0.5-mile trek rather than the same descent over less than half that distance along the blue trail.

Continue along the right fork, following white paints, about 0.25 mile, where you reach a small gully and a vantage point to see the seasonal falls along Spring Brook. My suspicion is that these falls run dry far sooner than the ones along Lick Brook, so you might want to plan a trip during the spring thaw to see water flowing here. The path winds westward, and you are soon traversing a ridge between two shallow valleys. The ridge is not much wider than the path itself, making an interesting passage beside the typically dry brook.

The trail takes a hard left turn at 0.65 mile; 0.1 mile farther, you reach the edge of the forest, above a clearing where railroad tracks cut a swath through the landscape. The trail turns back southward as you walk along a fairly flat portion of the trail. As you traverse this floodplain, you will likely notice some large sycamore trees whose smooth and peeling bark is markedly different than that of the typical hardwoods most often found throughout the Finger Lakes and Central New York.

After meandering less than 0.25 mile, you soon reconnect with Lick Brook and the blue trail back to the upper parking area. To reach the lower falls, you can easily rock-hop your way upstream to the basin below the falls. There is no pool at the base of the falls to speak of, but rather a steep limestone basin surrounds the verdant falls. Moss and vegetation climb along the gorge walls where the brook cascades 50 feet, and there is a broad, flat area to explore the amphitheater-like enclosure. Those with the urge to scale the gorge should note the sign warning that climbing the gorge walls is strictly prohibited without a permit from the Finger Lakes Land Trust.

At this point you can head back to the parking area, 0.6 mile away and a total round-trip of 1.6 miles. Alternatively you could take a side trip to Cayuga Inlet. The side trip is only 0.75 mile round-trip, extending your trip to approximately 2.4 miles total. Mostly a path through an open field, the side trip provides a welcome diversion from the woodland and an excellent opportunity to add some wildlife viewing to your hike. To reach the open field, head downstream, following white paints, and cross Lick Brook just past a small boulder with a memorial plaque set into it. The plaque commemorates Howard Edward Babcock, an innovator of modern farming techniques, noted Cornell University professor, and once chairman of Cornell's board of trustees. In 1997 Howard's son, John, donated a 27-acre parcel of land to Cornell. This land gift is now one of Cornell Plantations' nature preserves and abuts the Sweedler Preserve to the south.

Once out in the field, the trail paints are more difficult to find; there actually are some on small saplings, but the path is well worn through the high grass, so finding your way through this section is not too difficult. The worn path soon reaches Cayuga Inlet near a railroad bridge. The Finger Lakes Trail continues on the other side of Cayuga Inlet, but this is as good a point as any at which to turn around, so head back along the field path to the base of the lower falls.

Back near the base of the lower falls, follow the blue blazes uphill to return to the parking area along Town Line Road. The climb from this point onward is fairly steep at times. Recently, Cornell

Outdoor Education students have built several switchbacks to ease the vertical nature of the trail, but nevertheless the climb is steep. A short distance along the climb, you catch a glimpse of the middle falls along the brook. This 25-foot-tall waterfall is not far from the top of the lower falls, is more angular, and has a steeper vertical drop than the lower falls. You can view the falls from a small overlook on your right. Again use caution when approaching the edge of the cliff.

Continue uphill and eastward, following multiple switchbacks and steep sections. Along this climb, views of the ever-deepening gorge on your right are obscured by surrounding foliage, but as you near the reconnection with the FLT, you might catch a good view of the top of the upper falls previously mentioned. These are perhaps the safest points from which to view the upper falls, though in dry times and when the trees are leafed out, not much will be visible. Again extreme caution should be used near the edges. You reconnect with Finger Lakes Trail at 1.3 miles (roughly 2 miles if you took the side trip), and from here it is just another 0.25 mile back to the parking area along Town Line Road.

Directions

From the intersection of NY 79 and NY 13/NY 34 in Ithaca, continue south along NY 13/NY 34/NY 96/Elmira Road. Pass the entrance to Buttermilk Falls State Park, and take the first left onto Sand Bank Road, 400 feet past the park entrance. Follow Sand Bank Road along a sharp right turn and continue 1.6 miles. Bear right onto Town Line Road. The pulloff is less than 0.1 mile down Town Line Road. Look for the yellow Finger Lakes Trail signs and the large green Sweedler Preserve sign, just before the bridge crossing Lick Brook.

Connecticut Hill Wildlife Management Area: Bob Cameron Loop

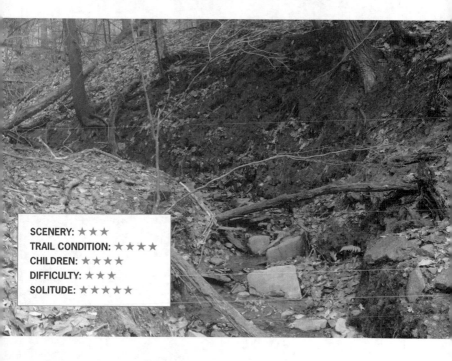

SCENERY: ★ ★ ★
TRAIL CONDITION: ★ ★ ★ ★
CHILDREN: ★ ★ ★ ★
DIFFICULTY: ★ ★
SOLITUDE: ★ ★ ★ ★ ★

GPS TRAILHEAD COORDINATES: N42° 23.144'   W76° 40.117'

DISTANCE & CONFIGURATION: 2.6-mile loop

HIKING TIME: 1–1.5 hours

HIGHLIGHTS: Quiet woodland, old foundation, passport trail

ELEVATION: 2,120' at trailhead; 1,720' at lowest point

ACCESS: Open 24/7; no fees or permits required

MAPS: FLT trail map: Sheet M16; DEC map: **dec.ny.gov/outdoor/55723.html**

FACILITIES: None

WHEELCHAIR ACCESS: No

COMMENTS: Wildlife management areas are very active during hunting season, so plan your trip accordingly.

CONTACTS: NYSDEC Regional Wildlife Manager, Region 7, 607-753-3095, ext. 247, **dec.ny.gov/outdoor/9331.html**

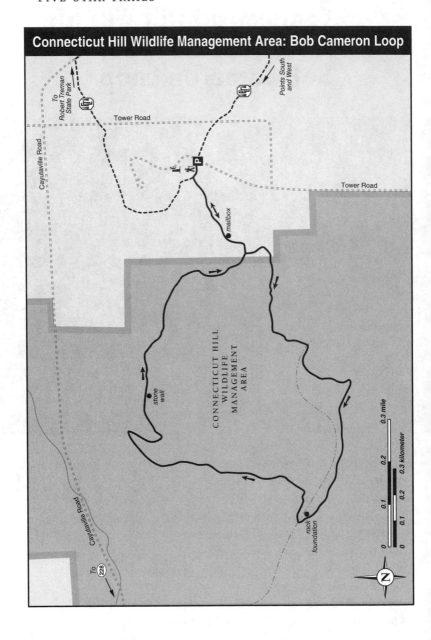

Connecticut Hill Wildlife Management Area: Bob Cameron Loop

Overview

This relatively straightforward loop through a quiet woodland is actually one of the highest points found within the Finger Lakes region. There are no panoramic vistas, but the trail has enhanced tributary crossings, an abandoned old homestead, and a bit of elevation change to add a little vigor to an otherwise flat region. Finger Lakes passport hikers will also have one more destination to cross off their list.

Route Details

The trailhead lies along the west side of the dirt road, a few hundred feet shy of the cell tower and across from a yellow Finger Lakes Trail (FLT) sign on the road's east side. The FLT bisects the road here on its way to Robert H. Treman State Park (see page 175 for a description of that trail). Counterintuitively, the white-blazed trail to your right that heads eastward connects with the southern portion of the Connecticut Hill Wildlife Management Area, while the trail to the left heads westward but is the eventual path to Robert H. Treman State Park, actually to the northeast. To reach the Bob Cameron Loop, head west along the former option, following white paints about a few hundred feet to an intersection. To the right, the white trail continues to Robert H. Treman State Park, while the left path, marked with orange paints, is the beginning of the Bob Cameron Loop.

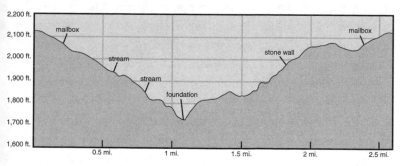

Head downhill and you soon pass a mailbox along the trail. The mailbox is one of 12 similar trail registers found scattered along the FLT system. The Finger Lakes passport program is a partnership between businesses and the Finger Lakes Trail Conference (FLTC) and is meant as an incentive to get people outdoors and enjoying a more active lifestyle. Participants in the program can take rubbings of the placards affixed to the mailbox posts to prove that they have hiked the trails. Participants who collect four or more rubbings are eligible for a special patch supplied by the FLTC. Details as well as a brochure describing the program are available at participating sponsors or online at **fltconference.org/trail/whats-happening/hike-programs/passport.**

The mailbox also has a normal trail register inside and is just a short distance before the beginning of the loop section of the trail. Bear left at the loop intersection and head south. The trail descends approximately 300 feet over the next 0.75 mile, crossing and recrossing a tributary stream of Cayuta Lake three times. You reach the first crossing about 0.25 mile ahead, and the rock-hop across will barely break your stride. The second crossing is a slightly more involved affair, where the banks of the stream are more deeply cut. Hemlocks crowd the stream at these crossings and give the area a more primeval feel.

Once across, the trail descends along the ridgeline above the gully that encompasses the stream. Dense carpets of ferns and club mosses line the hillside to your left. Club mosses are not true mosses and are often mistaken as small evergreen saplings, but their real nature is far more interesting. Sometimes referred to as ground pines or running pines, these evergreen perennials are ancient in nature. Their origins reach back to the Paleozoic era, more than 300 million years ago. Indeed, they have more in common with the ancient trees that made up the vast forest jungles blanketing the world when life first expanded onto the land than with the forests we see today. Their most prolific means of propagation is along running roots whose new stems grow into thick carpets, as seen to the side of the trail here. Similar to ferns (they are often referred to as fern allies), they also reproduce through spores. The microscopic spores were once an important part of commerce and had a wide variety of uses, ranging from microscopic measurement aids, ingredients for soothing ailments and coating pills, and even fireworks.

Soon you reach the bottom of a hill next to the stream, at 1.1 miles. On the right side of the trail near the stream crossing are an old rock foundation and metal pump, both most likely remnants of an old homestead present before 10,000 acres of land were purchased by the state soon after the beginning of the 20th century. The management area now encompasses more than 11,000 acres and is the largest wildlife management area in the state.

You are not quite halfway along the loop, but this is the best stopping point along the loop, if you are looking for one. Make your final rock-hop across the tributary stream, now much wider than before, and begin the climb back to the parking area.

The trail quickly bends to the north, and you climb gradually along an old logging road the next 0.5 mile until you encounter a sharp turn in the trail. Marked with an orange arrow, the trail turns sharply to the right and begins a much steeper ascent. Proceed up multiple small switchbacks. Approximately 0.25 mile along your ascent, you will pass through an old stone wall that bisects the trail and will briefly head into an old pine plantation. At 2.3 miles, you return to the panhandle portion of the trail at the passport mailbox. From here it is another 0.3 mile back to the parking area, for a total trip length of 2.6 miles.

Directions

Follow directions to Robert H. Treman State Park (page 175). Continue south past the park, and turn along NY 13 South/NY 34 South/NY 96/Elmira Road. Bear right to remain on NY 13 South/Elmira Road. Turn right onto CR 134/Millard Hill Road, at 1.1 miles. At 3.9 miles, take a slight left onto Connecticut Hill Road. After 1.2 miles, bear right to stay on Connecticut Hill Road for 0.9 mile. Turn right on Tower Road. The parking area is about 0.75 mile on your left, just before the cell tower.

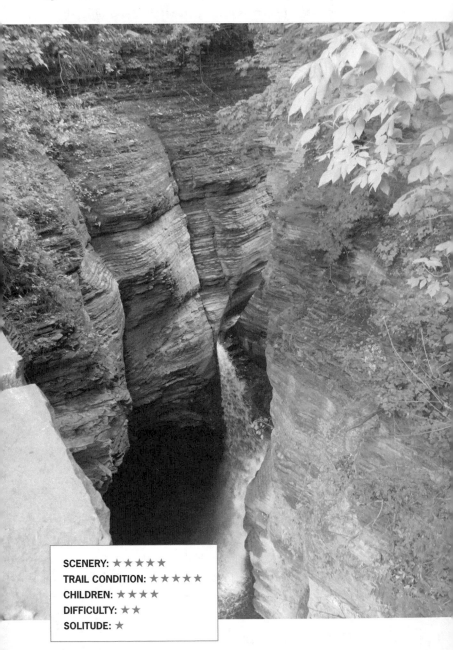

SCENERY: ★ ★ ★ ★ ★
TRAIL CONDITION: ★ ★ ★ ★ ★
CHILDREN: ★ ★ ★
DIFFICULTY: ★ ★
SOLITUDE: ★

GPS TRAILHEAD COORDINATES: N42° 22.499'   W76° 52.445'

DISTANCE & CONFIGURATION: 3.0-mile out-and-back along the Gorge Trail; 3.0-mile loop when combined with the North Rim Trail

HIKING TIME: 1–1.5 hours

HIGHLIGHTS: Scenic gorge, waterfalls, tunnels, elaborate stonework

ELEVATION: 490' at lower trailhead; 1,010' at upper trailhead

ACCESS: Daily, sunrise–sunset; the Gorge Trail is only open mid-May–early November; $8 vehicle entrance fee

MAPS: New York State Park map: **nysparks.com/parks/142/maps.aspx**; also available at entrance booth

FACILITIES: Restrooms, concessions, gift shop, picnic areas, shuttle

WHEELCHAIR ACCESS: No

COMMENTS: No dogs or alcoholic beverages allowed on the Gorge Trail.

CONTACTS: New York State Office of Parks, 607-535-4511, **nysparks.com/parks/142**

Overview

Watkins Glen is truly a spectacle of both natural beauty and trail construction. A plethora of waterfalls, potholes, plunge pools, flumes, and sheer cliffs alone make a visit to this gorge worthwhile. Add the carefully crafted stone staircases, bridges, walls, and tunnels, and this becomes a can't-miss excursion. The trail is definitely one of the more popular and congested trails featured in the book, but the scenery makes it well worth joining the crowds.

Route Details

Admittedly, my personal tastes for hiking trails tend more toward remote wilderness settings than anything you will find in Watkins Glen State Park. Indeed the park abuts a busy commercial street in the middle of the village of Watkins Glen. However, what nature and man have crafted within this gorge is truly a marvel and something any visitor to the region should experience at least once. Layers of ancient stone have been cut, sculpted, gouged, smoothed, and organically shaped by surging waters for millennia. This stonework alone has a natural poetry to it that could never be replicated by humans. But

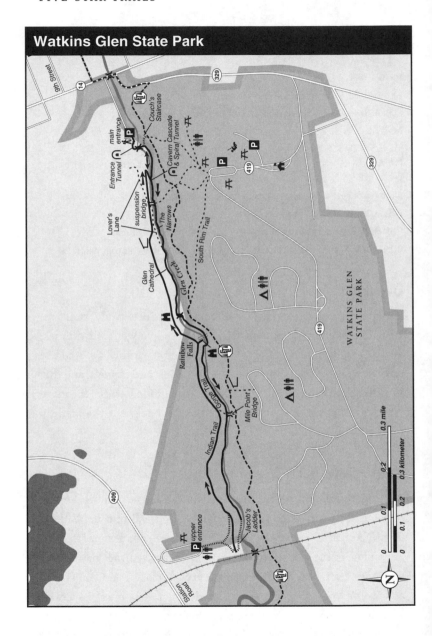

Watkins Glen State Park

I am also a craftsperson at heart, so I find equally impressive the marvels of stonework constructed beside, built into, and cut through the gorge. Complementing each other, the two blend together so well that it is often hard to discern where one begins and the other ends. It is one of those rare occurrences where the hand of humankind enhances the natural setting, and I have no doubt you'll agree.

Originally viewed as an obstruction to the pastoral ambitions of early settlers, the "glen" was relegated to industrial purposes. A large saw- and gristmill were located in what is presently the parking area, and additional mills were sited farther along the glen. An informal network of paths and wooden bridges delved ever deeper into the gorge, providing access to these mills. These paths were used by the first tourists to the glen when Judge George C. Freer opened the gorge in 1851. Morvalden Ells, a journalist from Elmira, was among the original tourists. He was so enraptured by the glen that he took on the principal role of promoting the gorge as a marvel of nature to rival Niagara Falls. His imaginative and often romantic descriptions of the glen created the beginning of a tourist trade that endures today. The glen remained under private development and supervision until the turn of the 20th century, when it was purchased by the state for $46,000. The original purchase included 103 acres and was administered by the American Scenic and Historic Preservation Society (ASHPS). It was at this point that the gorge began its transformation

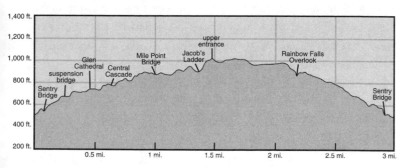

into what we see today. The transformation included removing the vestiges of its industrial past but, more important, removing the hazardous network of paths, wooden stairs, and bridges. Concrete, iron, and steel became the basis of the infrastructure, and great effort was expended in broadening the paths and tying the new bridges and iron guardrails into the gorge's walls. Workers were often lowered into the glen on slings to carry out the work along the steep walls, while blasting and tunneling took place elsewhere. The trail begins inside one of these hand-cut tunnels.

The aptly named Entrance Tunnel is hard to miss, and as you ascend the series of stairs, you begin to grasp the scope of the work done here. After emerging from the tunnel, you cross Sentry Bridge and first glimpse the natural wonders of the gorge. Below a small chute forms a surging waterfall, approximately 25 feet tall. The bridge gets quite congested, and you may only get to glimpse this waterfall in passing. Don't worry—there are more than enough waterscapes ahead. As you climb the stone stairs, you might notice that the iron handrails mentioned previously are, simply put, missing. Their absence—as well as the absence of concrete—marks the next step of the narrative as the glen has evolved into its present form.

In 1935 catastrophic floods washed away virtually all of the work done by the ASHPS. A Civilian Conservation Corps (CCC) crew, based in the park since the previous year, was suddenly transformed from a labor force into a rescue team as the town was inundated. Later the corps became a major force in the park's restoration and reconstruction. Although the floods were first seen as a tragedy, park designers soon believed them to be a blessing. Though the ASHPS had strived to build harmoniously with the landscape, bare iron and flat concrete were conspicuously industrial when compared with the naturally carved walls of the gorge. Instead, the new design would incorporate natural stone in the paths, staircases, and stone walls. The goal was to blend the construction into the landscape, and as you weave your way up through the glen, you can't help but admire how well they achieved that goal.

Continuing along the Gorge Trail, you soon pass a staircase that connects to the South Rim Trail (an alternative return route). The South Rim Trail is yet another section of the North Country Trail that passes by the Six Nations Campground, featured in the guidebook *Best Tent Camping: New York State*. A short distance past the staircase, your attention is drawn to Cavern Cascade looming ahead. One of two waterfalls that the trail passes behind, Cavern Cascade is another congestion point. Before ascending the stairs to the falls, take a moment to head down a different set of stairs to a viewing point lower down, near Glen Creek. Powerfully sculpted plunge pools riddle this portion of the creek, and the lower vantage point allows you to look back on the narrow gorge behind you, in addition to admiring the lower drop of Cascade Falls, which falls a total of 38 feet.

As you climb and approach the upper portion of Cascade Falls, you begin to see why congestion builds here. Everyone is taking pictures not only of the falls, with family members behind them, but also from behind the falls. You can hardly blame fellow sightseers; the falls are certainly picturesque, and looking back through the water will provide great pictures even if they're snapped in a hurry. The passage behind the falls is barely enough for two to shuffle past, so be mindful of how much time you spend.

To the delight of many, the passage behind the falls is followed by the Spiral Tunnel, where again we encounter the remnants of ASHPS construction. The wide spiral staircase adds a bit of mystery about what lies ahead, and you certainly won't be disappointed by the Narrows when you get there. Constricted and dark, the Narrows have a primeval feel, where mosses and ferns grow abundantly in the shady microclimate. As you pass through the Narrows, look up and you will see a suspension bridge overhead, 85 feet above you. Now consider that when the 1935 flood swept through this narrow chasm, that water surged within 5 feet of it. Imagine that surge of water as you pass an intersection with Lover's Lane, travel through another tunnel, and then climb up another set of stairs before entering into Glen Cathedral.

Wide and open, the Glen Cathedral has a drastically different feel from the Narrows. Sunlight is abundant, but sheer 200-foot-tall cliff walls limit the vegetation to this side of the flat stream. Ahead, the Central Cascade, 42 feet high, is wonderfully framed by a narrowing of the cliff walls, but also by a handsome stone bridge that arches over its 4-foot-wide crest. You climb a winding series of equally handsome stone steps and pass through another tunnel before you cross the bridge and enter into the Glen of Pools. A variety of potholes and plunge pools provides another marvelous example of water's sculpting power (see Buttermilk Falls State Park: Gorge Trail, page 157, for a description of this process). Ahead is one of the most iconic scenes along the gorge and another congestion point, so linger here a while if the trail has become crowded and you hope to experience the upcoming setting at a more leisurely pace.

More stone steps bring you to where the path passes under an arching mass of stone and Rainbow Falls. Ahead is another falls, this time the 12-foot-high cascade at Rainbow Falls, that passes under another arched stone bridge. The trail under the falls and up to the bridge is often slick and narrow, so mind your step as you pass. Once over the bridge, you are again on the north side of the ravine and will enter another aptly named section, the Spiral Gorge.

If you failed to notice the curving nature of some of the features along the creek, you will now. The hourglass-shaped sculpting is what remains when two neighboring potholes widen so much that they eventually blow out the dividing section of stone between them. The process of transformation of stream to plunge pool to pothole to sinuously sculptured stream was repeated over and over through this narrow passage. The path grows darker and narrower as you proceed to its conclusion by a series of flumes and chutes. Morvalden Ells named one of these Pluto Falls, after the Roman god of the underworld, a clear demonstration of Ells's flare for the dramatic when concocting names to enhance his romantic vision of the gorge.

Climb another stone staircase beneath an overhanging cliff and emerge from the gorge "underworld" out onto the uppermost

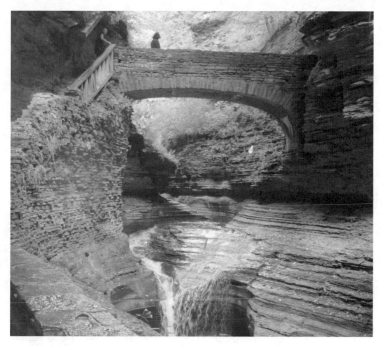

STONE BRIDGE

section of the gorge. A short way ahead lies Mile Point Bridge. Hard to believe, but you have traveled only a little more than a mile. There are no more dramatic flumes or waterfalls, only placid waters ahead. At the bridge you have multiple choices. First, you could cross the bridge and return via the South Rim Trail, which, as mentioned, connects to the campgrounds. Second, you could continue 0.5 mile farther along Glen Creek and climb 180 steps up Jacob's Ladder to the upper park area. From the upper entrance you can return via the shuttle bus or the Indian Trail along the north rim. Third and last, you could turn around and return the way you came. When I visited, I chose the Indian Trail, as I thought it had the greatest chance for lookouts down into the gorge. There are some, but they are mostly obscured until you reach the suspension bridge previously mentioned. The bridge connects the north and south rims, and you can return to the

Gorge Trail shortly after, to a point just before the Spiral Tunnel. For the sake of some solitude, I recommend returning along the north rim, but the best option for scenery is to return the way you came.

Nearby Attractions

Every fall, Watkins Glen becomes a hub for car-racing fans when the Watkins Glen International ("The Glen") races are held. Leading up to and following the races, campgrounds, hotels, and RV lots are full to capacity. Race fans have been coming since 1948, when the race featured a mixture of road surfaces along public roads. Since then, the course has undergone several revisions and changed locations to a private facility southwest of the village of Watkins Glen. More information, including the schedule for the current year's race, is available at **theglen.com.**

Directions

From Ithaca *(points east)*: Follow NY 79 West out of Ithaca. Follow NY 79 West for 21 miles, where, at the bottom of a steep hill, NY 79 West merges with NY 414 South. Follow NY 414 South into Watkins Glen, and, at 1.6 miles, turn left on NY 414 South/NY 14 South/North Franklin Street. The lower park entrance is 0.3 mile ahead on your right.

From Horseheads *(points south)*: From the intersections of NY 14 North/Westinghouse Road and Watkins Road/North Main Street, head north for 14.9 miles along NY 14 North/Watkins Road. Park entrance is on the left.

From Geneva *(points northwest):* From I-90, take Exit 42 (NY 14/ Geneva/Lyons). Merge onto NY 318 East, and turn right onto NY 14 South at 0.2 mile. Follow NY 14 South 5.9 miles into Geneva. Continue along NY 14 South for 35.8 miles into Watkins Glen. Park entrance is on your right.

27 Queen Catharine Marsh: Willow Walk

SCENERY: ★ ★ ★
TRAIL CONDITION: ★ ★ ★ ★
CHILDREN: ★ ★ ★ ★
DIFFICULTY: ★
SOLITUDE: ★ ★ ★ ★ ★

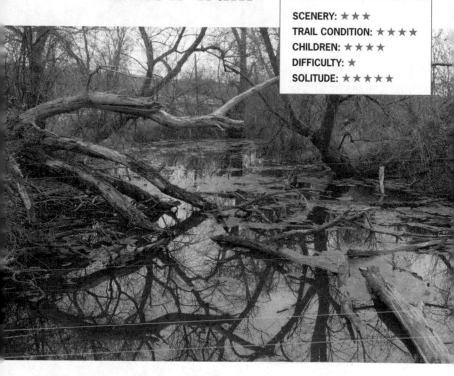

GPS TRAILHEAD COORDINATES: N42° 21.540'   W76° 50.466'

DISTANCE & CONFIGURATION: 2.0-mile loop

HIKING TIME: 1 hour

HIGHLIGHTS: Wetland, wildlife viewing, birding

ELEVATION: 458' at trailhead, with no significant rise

ACCESS: Open 24/7; no fees or permits required

MAPS: Finger Lakes Trail Conference: Sheet QCMLT; DEC Catharine Creek area map: dec.ny.gov/outdoor/31021.html

FACILITIES: None

WHEELCHAIR ACCESS: No

COMMENTS: A small section of the trail traverses a parking area and docks along the Chemung Barge Canal. This section can be avoided by returning the way you came or by following the abandoned airport road.

CONTACTS: DEC Region 8, 585-226-2466, dec.ny.gov/outdoor/24429.html

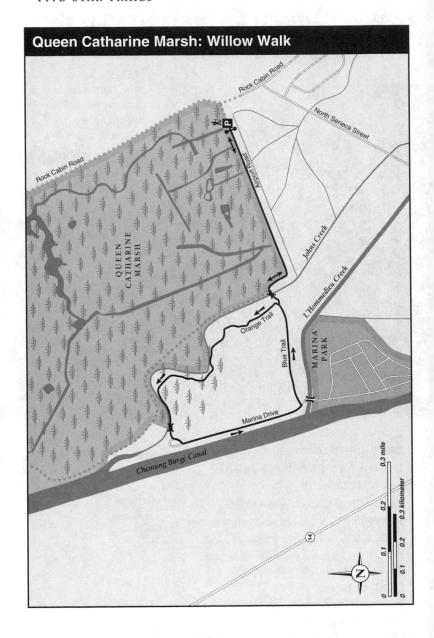

Queen Catharine Marsh: Willow Walk

Overview

This short trek amid the marshland south of Seneca Lake is not particularly challenging but provides quiet hikers with some truly excellent opportunities to view wildlife. Birders can spot more than 64 species through the seasons, while fishermen will find the waters prime for 29 species of fish. The ease of the trail and ample wildlife make for an excellent opportunity to introduce new hikers—both young and old—to the pleasure of the outdoors.

Route Details

Willow Walk passes through a small section of a 1,000-acre marshland that has served the Watkins Glen area for a variety of purposes, from fur trapping and agriculture to an industrial canal and even an airport runway. Today it serves as one of the last remaining headwater marshes and is an important habitat, especially for birds that require an aquatic environment. Although technically called the Catharine Creek Fish and Wildlife Management Area, it is simply known as Queen Catharine Marsh. Odds are that you will have guessed the area was named after a British monarch during the Colonial period. Well, you would be half correct. The name does derive from the Colonial era, but the namesake was a local Seneca Indian queen, Catharine Montour. Little is actually known about this "queen" except that she was a leader of a village of approximately 300 Seneca Indians who lived on the south shore of Seneca Lake in what is today Watkins Glen and Montour Falls. When the American Sullivan-Clinton expedition raided the area in an attempt to drive out all British-allied American Indians, Catharine and her villagers are reported to have fled for Fort Niagara in Canada. She is believed to have died in 1804, but whether it was in Canada or back in Montour Falls is disputed. Nevertheless her moniker is still widely used in the area.

To begin the trail, head westward, past the vehicle barrier gate, and along the old airport access road. As expected, the road is broad, flat, and free of obstruction, allowing you to view the expanse of marshland sprawling to the north. You cross multiple channels that weave through the grasslands to the north and feed from the wetland forest to the south (to your left). Orange paints mark the way, though finding the path is effortless. You will make quick time along this stretch and soon reach a point where the road bends to the right, heading north. After this turn, keep an eye out for the footpath off to your left, marked by an orange arrow. Turn left and head westward across a wooden bridge into dense scrubs and undergrowth. The trail narrows and you quickly reach a trail intersection at just shy of 0.5 mile. Ahead is a blue trail—and probable return leg, described later on. To your right is the continuation of the orange trail and our path onward. As you head northward along the orange-marked trail, the scrub and underbrush grow so thick that it limits your views. As opposed to the open expanse along the access road, this area has a more closed-in feel. At first I disliked the dramatic change, but I soon came to appreciate that the dense cover allows hikers to sneak up on the ample wildlife in the region. Birdsong becomes appreciably louder, and squirrels and chipmunks scurry about everywhere. Tread softly and you will have an even better chance to see more interesting wildlife. On my excursion, great blue herons seemed to be around every corner and could be found fishing in numerous places along the meandering creek that weaves through the area. Many worn paths lead down to this log-strewn and verdant creek, providing many interesting places to view scenes where wildlife tends to congregate.

Just under 1 mile from the trailhead, you will reach a fork in the trail. A wooden bridge leads off to the right, while the main trail continues straight ahead through an opening in a dense hedgerow. Across the bridge is a broad, open field that leads back toward the open marshland. The old airport road is also across this bridge and could provide a different route back to the trailhead. At this point you will have to make a choice: Follow the prescribed route or head back the way you came. In all honesty, returning the way you came is likely the most scenic option. However, I've always preferred loops, so I'll describe the designated loop for those who, like me, are sticklers for

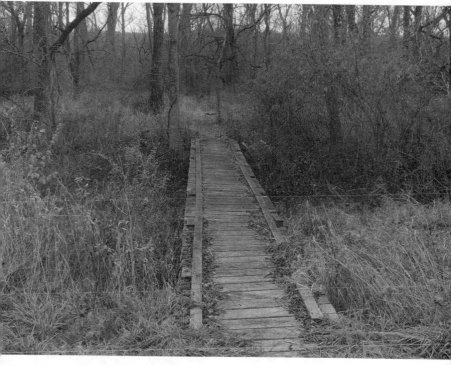

QUEEN CATHARINE MARSH BRIDGE

not retracing their steps when given a choice. To follow the designated loop, continue straight through the hedgerow out onto Marina Drive. This road is primarily an access road to the many boat slips along the old Chemung Barge Canal. Just in case you want reassurance that you are indeed along the designated path, there are orange paints along many of the utility poles that line the drive. Bear left and continue south along the road a little over 0.25 mile past the numerous boat slips, tents, and picnic areas. Once you reach the steel-grate bridge that crosses L'Hommedieu Creek, turn left up a small hill and onto a short berm. The trail, marked in blue, follows the top of this berm briefly but soon winds down into the surrounding woodland. The trail continues east, briefly running beside one of the many branches of Seneca Lake Inlet and then returning to the fork (along the loop previously encountered) approximately 1.5 miles from the start. Continue east back to the old airport road and follow your path back to the parking area along Rock Cabin Road for a total trip length of just over 2 miles.

Nearby Attractions

Willow Walk is just a short portion of a longer historic walk that circuits the marsh and sections of Watkins Glen. The Queen Catharine Marsh loop (8.1 miles) mostly follows the roads that encircle the marsh, with a small portion along what would properly be termed a trail (that which is featured here). This longer circuit is similar to the Montour Falls Historic loop (5.5 miles) in that both are rather civilized, run mostly along roads, and are not necessarily trails. Maps for both of these walks are available from the Finger Lakes Trail Conference at **fltconference.org.** Similar in nature to and actually adjoining these trails is the 12-mile one-way multiuse Catharine Valley Trail (CVT). This trail follows much of the abandoned towpath along the Chemung Barge Canal and the Pennsylvania Railroad, but is probably more to the tastes of cyclists than hikers seeking a wilderness experience. The multiuse trail is part of the New York state parks system; information is available at **nysparks.com/parks/80/details.aspx.**

Directions

From NY 14/Catharine Street in Montour Falls, turn onto NY 224/Clawson Boulevard. Follow it eastward 0.5 mile and take your third left onto North L'Hommedieu/CR 8. The sharp turn is at the bottom of a steep hill along NY 224, so if you begin to climb, you have gone too far. Bear left onto Rock Cabin Road 0.4 mile ahead. Take the third left onto Airport Road, at 0.3 mile. Parking is on the right side of the road just before the vehicle barrier gate.

Connecticut Hill Wild-life Management Area: Cayuta Creek

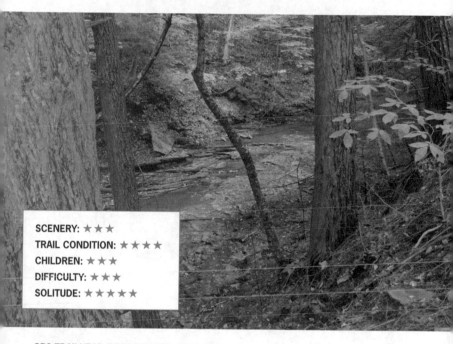

SCENERY: ★ ★ ★
TRAIL CONDITION: ★ ★ ★ ★
CHILDREN: ★ ★ ★
DIFFICULTY: ★ ★ ★
SOLITUDE: ★ ★ ★ ★ ★

GPS TRAILHEAD COORDINATES: N42° 20.970' W76° 44.234'

DISTANCE & CONFIGURATION: 5.7-mile loop

HIKING TIME: 3–4 hours

HIGHLIGHTS: Creek-side stroll, quiet woodland

ELEVATION: 1,318' at trailhead; 1,700' at highest point along loop

ACCESS: Open 24/7; no fees or permits required

MAPS: Finger Lakes Trail Conference: Sheet M16; DEC map: **dec.ny.gov/outdoor /55723.html**

FACILITIES: None

WHEELCHAIR ACCESS: No

COMMENTS: Wildlife management areas are very active during hunting season, so plan your trip accordingly.

CONTACTS: NYSDEC Regional Wildlife Manager, Region 7, 607-753-3095 ext. 247, **dec.ny.gov/outdoor/9331.html**

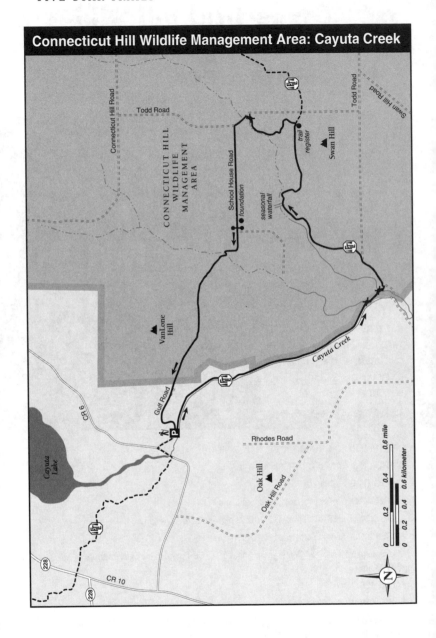

Connecticut Hill Wildlife Management Area: Cayuta Creek

Overview

The trail described is sometimes referred to as the Van Lone Hill Trail Loop and begins along a relatively flat section along the North Country Trail/Finger Lakes Trail (FLT) but also includes some moderate climbs and varied terrain farther along. A few sections of rustic roads help to complete the loop.

Route Details

From the pulloff on the west side of Gulf Road, head southeast past the Barton Dam memorial plaque and boulder. The trailhead is marked with white paints and a yellow Finger Lakes Trail sign. The trail here is a pleasant broad gravel path that follows Cayuta Creek as it flows southeast to the Susquehanna River. The creek is the outlet of Cayuta Lake, less than a mile north of the trailhead, and flows 35.2 miles southeast, until it empties into the Susquehanna River just past the New York–Pennsylvania border. Eventually these waters will empty into the Chesapeake Bay in Maryland, but we will only accompany them approximately 1.5 miles. Along this stroll, the white-blazed trail follows a relatively flat grade. The surrounding forest heavily shades the trail, which is in such good condition that you can easily look out and observe the creek without worrying about a root or other obstruction catching your feet. If you are lucky

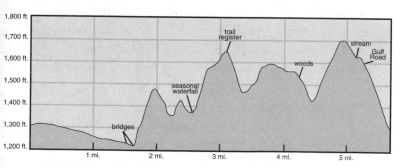

enough, you might even spot some interesting wildlife found in the area, including mink, muskrat, and various waterfowl. The 10,000-acre wildlife preserve was acquired shortly after the turn of the 20th century, and many studies and experimental programs have been conducted precisely to attract these types of wildlife to the area.

At roughly 1.5 miles, you reach the first of two bridges designed and built by the Cornell University student chapter of the American Society of Civil Engineers in conjunction with the Cayuga Trails Club. Installed in 2000, these heavy timber bridges, which are stout and narrow with tall guardrails, cross small tributaries of Cayuta Creek. After you cross the first bridge, the trail turns to your right, southward, where it narrows and begins to take on a more rugged character. You soon reach an intersection with a steep, rocky road coming downhill on your left. Bear right at this intersection, but then almost immediately turn left back onto the footpath. Do not follow the road. The trail continues essentially straight ahead here, but the bisecting road creates a small zigzag in the trail that is easy to overlook. Double paints indicate where the turns are, and you should stay on the footpath, as opposed to the broad road, and head slightly downhill into the small creek delta ahead. Continue to follow the white paints through this little delta to the second bridge crossing.

The bridge is nearly identical to the last one, and once across the bridge the trail begins to climb. After a short switchback, the trail intersects another abandoned forest road, about 0.1 mile from the last bridge, at 1.7 miles total. Turn north, to your left, and follow this hemlock-lined road uphill. The trail climbs approximately 150 feet over the next 0.25 mile, until it diverts to your left away from the road. It's easy to miss the turnoff, so keep an eye out for the double white paints indicating the slight turn.

The trail continues generally northward through a wet area among a stand of evergreens and then begins to wind its way downhill. At 2.5 miles, you near the end of your descent and enter into a hemlock grove that follows along the top of a gully. A primeval feel pervades the area, as you head eastward along the edge of the seasonal stream. It is an excellent spot to stop, though practically speaking you are not quite halfway. No doubt thru-hikers along the FLT agree with the choice of stopping points, as is evidenced by the abandoned campfire site found shortly ahead. However, if you do plan to stop, I recommend that you continue a little farther along, about 0.1 mile, to where a feeder stream falls over a sheer rock wall into this seasonal stream. In the height of summer this waterfall is likely dry, but in the spring or after heavy rains, your rest stop could be accompanied by the sounds of falling water.

The trail turns southward, to your right, and heads uphill and away from this little hemlock grove shortly after passing the seasonal waterfall. The forest is a little more mature than previously encountered, with some very large trees shading the trail as you climb steadily over the next 0.5 mile, roughly 200 feet of elevation gain. Approximately 0.25 mile along this climb, you intersect an abandoned road on your right and then farther on reach the trail register near the end of the climb, at a little more than 3 miles total. At the trail register there is a fork in the trail; the white Finger Lakes Trail continues straight ahead farther into the Connecticut Hill Wildlife Management Area, while our route, to the left, follows orange blazes to the north.

The trail begins to descend through a series of switchbacks approximately 0.25 mile to join the stream we left earlier. Continue upstream along the southern bank to the northeast another 0.25 mile, where, after crossing a narrow wooden bridge, you intersect Todd Road. Turn left on Todd Road (though no signs indicate the road name), cross over the stream we have been following, and then continue uphill along Todd Road. The orange paints marking the trail are hard to see amid the overgrown brush beside the road, but if you look hard in both directions, you can make them out. The road climbs steeply and then reaches an intersection. Double orange paints and an arrow—the first clearly visible indication you are still on the designated trail—show the trail continuing to the left, along the unmarked School House Road. Many trails in the Finger Lakes utilize roads to create loops, which

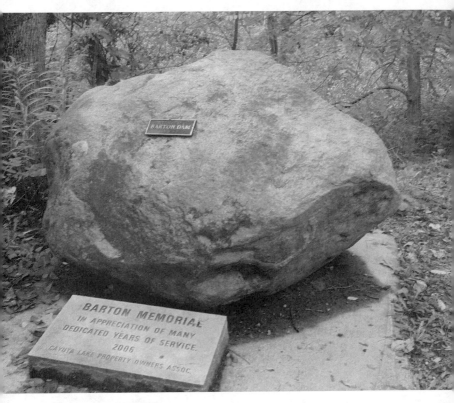

MEMORIAL BOULDER

I have to admit is not my favorite strategy to create appealing trails. In some circumstances the roads are heavily traveled, while in others, as is the case here, the roads are barely used, so they do preserve the wilderness setting sought by hikers. Unfortunately for me, I visited this trail on what must have been days after the roads had been regraded and shortly after heavy rains. The combination of the two converted what should have been an easy stroll into one long trek through slick clay and sucking mud. It is perhaps the only occasion on which I made worse time along a road than on a trail, and I spent the entire 0.5 mile slogging along as if my boots had suction cups. I have no doubt that the conditions have improved since, but it was an odd experience to say the least.

Again, trail markers along this portion are hard to make out through the overgrown brush, but you should continue almost 0.6 mile due east, past a small pulloff on your left where an old foundation is visible. Shortly after the foundation, the road takes a sharp left turn southward. At this point, the trail continues straight ahead and past some large boulders, where the orange paints are more visible. Follow the trail downhill to a small clearing and stream crossing, at 4.4 miles overall. Once across the stream, the trail bears to the right briefly and then begins a climb of 250 feet over the next 0.5 mile. Approximately 0.3 mile along the climb (4.7 miles overall), you intersect a road on your left. This is actually the first road that you crossed between the two bridges previously mentioned. The crest of your climb culminates among some pine trees, and though this is actually the highest point along the trip, it is doubtful you will notice. The descent back to your car, 0.8 mile ahead, is mostly uneventful, and you know you are getting close when you reach the end of the trail proper at 5.2 miles and begin the final 0.5-mile leg west along Gulf Road. The road takes a wide turn along its bend just before the parking lot comes into view for a round-trip length of 5.7 miles.

Directions

From the intersection of NY 13 and NY 224 in Cayuta, head north along NY 224 North for 3.5 miles, and turn right on CR 10. Follow CR 10 north 1.6 miles and turn right on CR 6, after 1.6 miles. Take a sharp right onto Gulf Road after 1 mile. Head 0.1 mile down Gulf Road to the small pulloff just before a large boulder and the yellow Finger Lakes Trail sign. The parking area has room for two or three cars, and the boulder has a memorial plaque for Barton Dam.

Shindagin Hollow State Forest

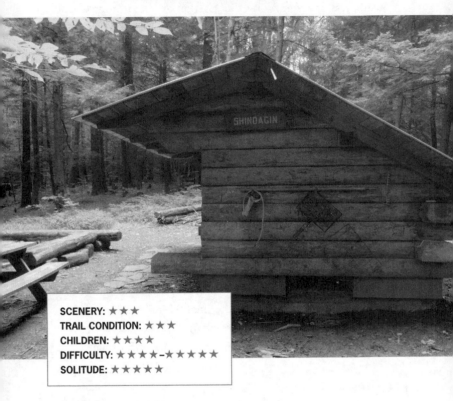

SCENERY: ★ ★ ★
TRAIL CONDITION: ★ ★ ★
CHILDREN: ★ ★ ★ ★
DIFFICULTY: ★ ★ ★ ★ – ★ ★ ★ ★ ★
SOLITUDE: ★ ★ ★ ★ ★

GPS TRAILHEAD COORDINATES: N42° 19.829'   W76° 21.055'

DISTANCE & CONFIGURATION: 6.2-mile out-and-back; 6.9-mile figure eight using roads

HIKING TIME: 2.5–3.5 hours

HIGHLIGHTS: Quiet woodland, streamside stroll, small waterfalls, scenic gorge, forest art

ELEVATION: 1,525' at trailhead; 1,717' at highest point along trail

ACCESS: Open 24/7; no fees or permits required

MAPS: Finger Lakes Trail Conference: Sheet M18; DEC Danby State Forest Map: **dec.ny
.gov/lands/64136.html**

FACILITIES: None

WHEELCHAIR ACCESS: No

COMMENTS: Normally I would not recommend for kids a 6.9-mile trail with as many ups and
downs as you'll find along the Shindagin Hollow loop. However, a couple of surprises along the

route will no doubt spark a youthful imagination, add some fun, and provide a unique experience. I'll leave the surprises for both young and older to discover. Nonetheless, I would not advise this trip for kids without proven stamina and a solid interest in hiking.

CONTACTS: Division of Lands & Forests, 607-753-3095, **dec.ny.gov/lands/64136.html**

Overview

Shindagin Hollow is a favorite spot for mountain bikers. However, their tracks and the hiking trails seldom share the same route. Even if the parking areas seem full, few of the visitors will actually be found along the hiking trails. Hiked either as a loop or an out-and-back, this trail has a lot of climbs and descents and is a great choice for hikers wanting a little more of a challenge compared to other trails in the region.

Route Details

From the ample parking area along Braley Hill Road, head a short distance south along the road to the Finger Lakes Trail (FLT). Turn left, and follow the white blazes of the FLT east to the trail register. The trail swings northward and soon intersects a blue-marked mountain biking trail and crosses a seasonal stream. After crossing the streambed, the trail immediately turns east and shortly after re-intersects the mountain biking trail, crosses the main branch of the same stream, and passes by a fire pit and camping area. Less than 0.25 mile ahead, the trail takes a series of sharp turns and soon reaches yet another intersection with the mountain biking trail network. This intersection is at an old forest road and will be the point you return to after completing the figure eight.

Continue straight over a small rock wall, following the blue- and white-marked FLT/North Country Trail (NCT), and begin a short descent of 150 feet over the next 0.25 mile. A short way along the descent, you'll cross a second wider forest road, after which the trail swings south and follows the contours of the hillside. Old stone foundations and walls are scattered to either side as you ease your way down until the trail swings east again and the descent grows

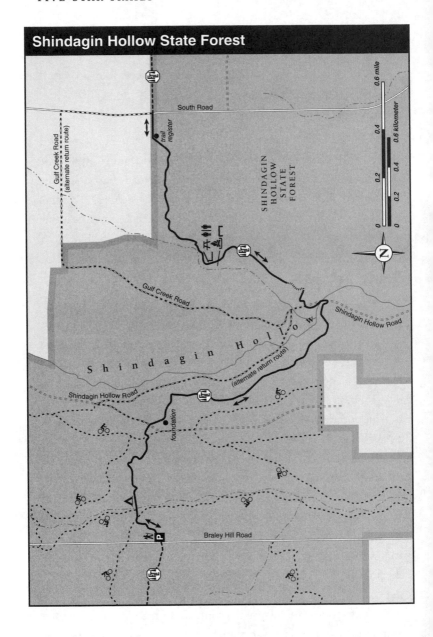

Shindagin Hollow State Forest

steeper, roughly 100 feet over 0.1 mile. The descent ends abruptly just before the much steeper slopes of Shindagin Hollow.

The trail turns sharply right and begins to regain much of its elevation loss as you follow the hollow's rim southward. After climbing for 0.25 mile, the trail reaches the crest, at a little over 1 mile overall, and then immediately begins a 325-foot descent over the next 0.75 mile down into Shindagin Hollow. The trail begins to level off where you cross through a wet area over wooden planks, and then it winds easterly to Shindagin Hollow Road. The path makes one last southward bend as it passes through a small hemlock knoll, and then crosses the roadside ditch along a short wooden bridge. This part of Shindagin Hollow Road offers alternative parking areas along the shoulder, as well as a little farther north near where Gulf Creek Road intersects Shindagin Hollow Road at a sharp turn in the road.

Turn left and follow the road northward very briefly to where the trail heads back into the woods on your left. This brief diversion weaves through an old orchard but quickly returns to Shindagin Hollow Road a little less than 300 feet farther from the point at which you left the road. Directly across the road is a newly built wooden bridge that crosses a small tributary creek. To your left you can see where the figure eight returns along Gulf Creek Road.

Once across the bridge, the trail heads mostly east along a forest road and fairly level ground until you reach a switchback built with

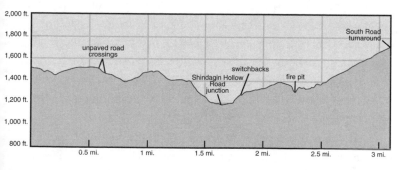

stone stairs. From this point forward the trail climbs out of Shindagin Hollow, gaining roughly 550 feet in elevation over the next 1.5
miles. In less than 0.1 mile, the trail re-intersects the washed-out forest road. Bear left and climb 0.25 mile along the forest road to where
the trail departs the road and heads westward toward a hemlock-
shrouded gully. As the Shindagin lean-to roof becomes visible on
your right, keep an eye out for a bench and fire pit located downhill
beside the gully. This little peninsula juts out into the deep gully and
would make an excellent alternative place to sit and rest if the other
spots by the lean-to are occupied. The area surrounding the lean-to
has many open spots and improvised benches that backpackers and
thru-hikers have obviously used in addition to the lean-to fire pit and
benches. It is obvious why this place, nestled along the side of the
wild gorge, is a popular destination.

Past the lean-to, the white-marked trail continues to hug the
gorge's rim, and soon a small cascade comes into view. The trail dips
in and out of several rivulets that feed the gorge for a little ways,
after which the trail veers right and begins to climb out of the hemlock forest. For the next 0.75 mile the trail climbs northeast toward
South Road through a typical deciduous forest. However, along the
climb you pass a remarkably atypical sight. This is the first of two
surprises found along the route forward. The second is encountered
farther ahead as the trail passes through a cedar grove and into a
clearing where the surprise and a passport mailbox await. (For more
about passport hikes, see the Connecticut Hill Wildlife Management
Area: Bob Cameron Loop on page 189.) From this clearing, you'll
pass through some more cedar groves, crossing seasonal streams,
and soon reach another trail register at 3.1 miles. From the register,
it is just a short way to South Road and the highest point along the
route (1,717 feet).

At this point you have two options: Return the way you came
or follow a series of roads back to Shindagin Hollow Road. Either
route you choose will involve a descent into the hollow before you
climb out again. The route back along the roads is mostly uneventful,

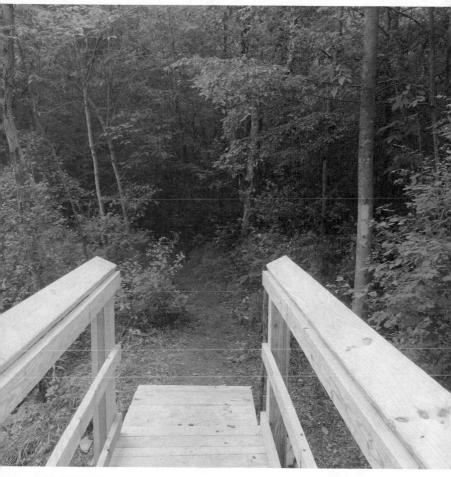

SHINDAGIN BRIDGE

but if you hate retracing your path as I do, I've outlined the route with mileage below.

Figure eight option along road network: Follow South Road 0.3 mile north to the Gulf Creek Road intersection; turn left on the gravel Gulf Creek Road. Follow it due west about 0.6 mile to a sharp left turn along Gulf Creek Road, and reenter Shindagin Hollow State Forest. After another 0.3 mile, the road sharply descends (325 feet along 0.75 mile) to the intersection with Shindagin Hollow Road. Turn right on Shindagin Hollow Road, follow it northwest past the wetland on your right, and begin climbing along Shindagin Hollow Road. Climb 300 feet over the next 0.75 mile and reach a point where the road levels off slightly. Yellow arrows are on the trees to your right, and a parking area for a handful of cars lies just ahead. The trail back to the Braley Hill Road parking area is almost directly behind you. First follow the forest road/mountain biking trail uphill to the FLT/NCT intersection at the rock wall you previously crossed. Turn right onto FLT/NCT, and follow it back to the parking area along Braley Hill Road for a round-trip of 6.9 miles.

Directions

From Ithaca, take NY 79 East/Slaterville Road east roughly 6.5 miles. Turn right onto CR 114/Boiceville Road, and follow it 0.6 mile; turn left onto CR 115/Central Chapel Road. Follow it south 2.6 miles, and then turn right onto Braley Hill Road. The parking area will be 1.5 miles on the left just before the FLT signs.

Danby State Forest: Abbott Hill Loop

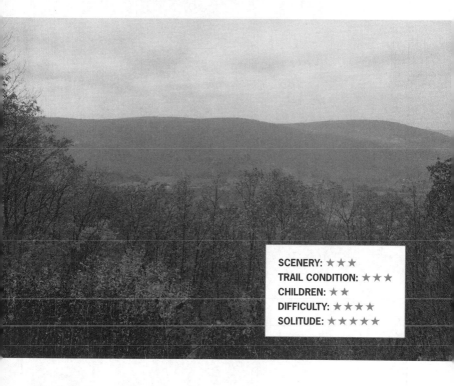

SCENERY: ★ ★ ★
TRAIL CONDITION: ★ ★ ★
CHILDREN: ★ ★
DIFFICULTY: ★ ★ ★ ★
SOLITUDE: ★ ★ ★ ★ ★

GPS TRAILHEAD COORDINATES: N42° 19.030'   W76° 28.670'

DISTANCE & CONFIGURATION: 8.3-mile loop

HIKING TIME: 4–5 hours

HIGHLIGHTS: Quiet woodland, streamside stroll, panoramic view

ELEVATION: 1,275' at trailhead; 1,716' at highest point along loop

ACCESS: Open 24/7; no fees or permits required

MAPS: Finger Lakes Trail Conference: Sheet Abbott Loop Trail; DEC Danby State Forest map: **dec.ny.gov/lands/64141.html**

FACILITIES: None

WHEELCHAIR ACCESS: No

COMMENTS: State forests are very active during hunting season, so plan your trip accordingly.

CONTACTS: Division of Lands & Forests, 607-753-3095, **dec.ny.gov/lands/64131.html**

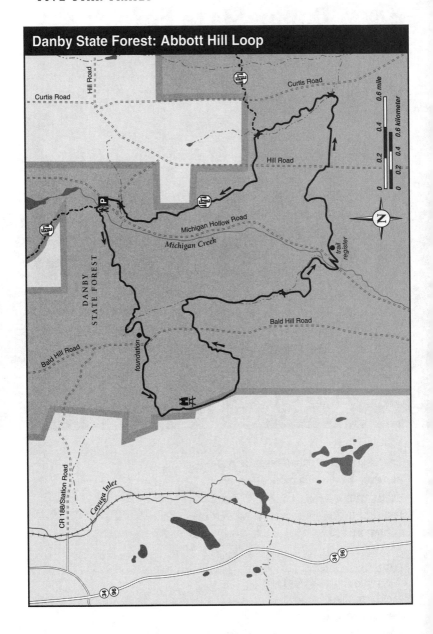

Danby State Forest: Abbott Hill Loop

Overview

With lots of climbs and descents, as well as a variety of different woodland environments, Abbott Hill Loop provides a great excursion for hikers who want to stretch their legs a bit. Long loops are rare in the region, and outdoor enthusiasts will delight in the seclusion furnished by this spread-out trail. Additionally, a panoramic view of the surrounding hills at Thatcher's Pinnacles provides another feature missing from other woodland trails in the region.

Route Details

The trail begins on the western side of Michigan Hollow Road. Proceed northeast, following the white-blazed Finger Lakes Trail (FLT), and cross a wooden bridge that spans Michigan Creek. Soon after crossing the meandering creek, the trail intersects the orange-marked Abbott Hill Loop on your left, a few hundred feet from Michigan Hollow Road. The trail heads generally westward and climbs steadily 200 feet over the next 0.5 mile. You'll pass a few old logging roads as you climb out of this valley, and just as the trail reaches the apex of the climb, it begins a winding course downhill to the west fork of Michigan Creek. The trail briefly parallels this creek northward but soon crosses the creek around the 1-mile mark. Once across, the trail switches back southward and climbs to a small ridge that follows the

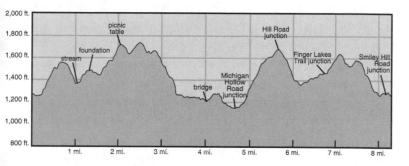

creek downstream. Follow this ridge a short way to where the trail swings westward, leaving the ridge behind. Just before intersecting Bald Hill Road, you pass by an abandoned foundation beside the trail, at 1.3 miles. Bear right onto the road and briefly follow it northwest to where the trail turns left and reenters the forest.

The trail immediately starts another 200-foot climb along a broad forest road for the next 0.5 mile. The ascent begins heading westward, but as the trail swings south, you near the top of the climb. Once you're around the corner, a clearing with a picnic table comes into view. You are now 2 miles along the trail and at Thatcher's Pinnacles. The forest is cleared around the picnic table, as well as along the steep hillside, and that clearing presents panoramic views westward of neighboring valleys and smooth ridges, characteristic of the region. These vistas are rare amid the heavily forested hilltops, and I am grateful that trail crews added this feature.

The U-shaped valley sprawling out before you is a result of the amazing scouring force that the Pleistocene glaciers exerted on the area. Typically valleys are created through erosion by either a stream or river, and the depth of the valley usually reflects the magnitude of such a water source. Note that despite the broad distance between ridges, there is no river or other body of water present that could account for such a broadly cut and flat depression between hillsides. Furthermore, the slopes are oddly steep along their sides but gently sloped at the ends. The hills—indeed nearly all hills within the Central New York and Finger Lakes region—are oriented along a north-south axis, yet another indication of the direction that ice flowed through the region. The awesome force that ice exerted in sculpting the modern landscape soon becomes very clear.

Continue south along this ridgeline about 0.25 mile to where the trail veers sharply to the left. This marks the corner of a private-property boundary marked by a yellow-painted stone marker. You continue southward as you climb to the highest elevation along the trail, 1,716 feet. Enter into mixed pines as you head eastward and soon after begin a 0.75-mile descent of 400 feet. Most of the gradual slope northeast stays beside the pines to your left, with hardwoods off to your right. You re-intersect and cross Bald Hill Road, about 0.5 mile along the descent, at nearly 3 miles total. Cross the road and continue to descend another 0.25 mile to the trail's reconnection with the western branch of Michigan Creek.

The trail turns southward and follows the streambed, weaving from one side to the other along a 0.6-mile stretch southward. You are now inside Bald Glen, and many sections along the creek are muddy with numerous downed trees, but trail crews have diligently cut through these obstructions. A quarter mile along this stroll southward within the creek bed, the trail crosses to the east of the creek and climbs onto an old logging road. The trail continues to follow the creek south, but you are now roughly 10–15 feet above it. The trail crosses the creek one more time along a log-and-plank bridge, 3.9 miles from the trailhead. From here the trail and stream diverge, and you begin a short climb southwest. The trail soon begins a broad curve back toward the creek, and you follow an elevated ridge, heavily shaded by hemlocks, to the southeast. The creek is again on your left, but you are dozens of feet above it.

At 4.4 miles, you begin to descend from this terrace and soon reach stream level near where the west and east branches of Michigan Creek converge. The trail bends to your right, southwest, around this confluence and briefly weaves through its delta before re-intersecting with Michigan Hollow Road. Turn left onto the road and follow it northeast over a broad culvert that crosses Michigan Creek. Rejoin the trail on the other side of the road just past the culvert.

The trail follows the creek very briefly and then turns left, northeast, and parallels the road a short distance. Just past a rocky outwash, you climb over a small hillock and reach a trail register; you're at 4.75 miles overall, about the midpoint of the circuit. Past the trail register, the trail makes a long climb eastward, 250 feet over 0.75 mile. The climb is mostly along old logging roads, but an occasional diversion off and back onto these roads occurs in a couple of spots before intersecting the heavily worn Hill Road at the top of the climb. The diversions

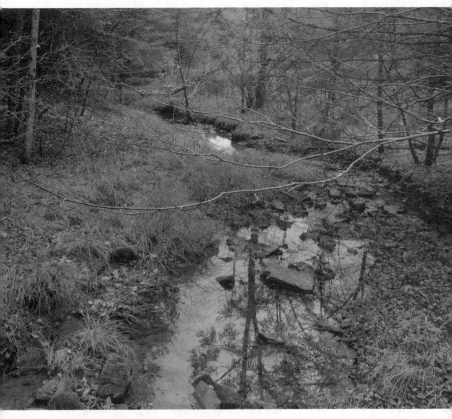

DANBY FORK ALONG MICHIGAN CREEK

include sharp turns, so keep an eye out for the double paints, and you should be able to navigate these small detours.

When you reach Hill Road—distinct from other forest roads by its worn and used surface—turn right and follow it briefly southward. The trail takes a sharp left off of Hill Road just before a fork along the main road. The trail begins to make an almost due-east descent of 300 feet over the next 0.5 mile. Along this descent the trail jogs around a rotten beech tree and joins a wider logging road heading down on your right. The orange paints are not immediately obvious here, but the road is. As you reach the end of your descent, you cross a series of wet areas along log-and-plank boardwalks, followed by a bridge over a tributary stream of Miller Creek, at 6.1 miles.

Across this bridge you begin to make your way northward, paralleling this stream up a gentle incline. Cross over another wet area along winding narrow log-and-plank boardwalks and, shortly after, intersect the FLT at a handsome wood sign. You have completed 6.6 miles so far and will follow the white-blazed FLT 1.7 miles for the remainder of the trip. Turn left and enter into an opening in the forest. You recross the stream you have been following north atop an old beaver dam and short wood bridges. Less than 0.25 mile ahead, you recross Hill Road. After climbing briefly eastward, the trail soon swings north and begins a long descent to Michigan Hollow Road. Most of the remaining trek north follows the contours of Michigan Hollow's eastern ridge. It is relatively uneventful unless you visit in late fall or winter, when you can see down into the hollow and across to the opposing ridge. Just before you return to the trailhead and your car, you veer briefly away from Michigan Hollow Road and cross a short wood bridge, a seasonal dirt road, and another short bridge, and then pass over a hillock and finally go down a steep hill back to Michigan Hollow Road for a round-trip of 8.3 miles.

Directions

From the intersection of Prospect Street/NY 96B and South Aurora Street in Ithaca, turn onto South Aurora Street/NY 96B heading south. After 0.5 mile, South Aurora Street/NY 96B becomes NY 96B/Danby Road. Turn right onto Michigan Hollow Road after 5.8 miles. Continue 2.4 miles south to the large parking pulloff on the west side of Michigan Hollow Road.

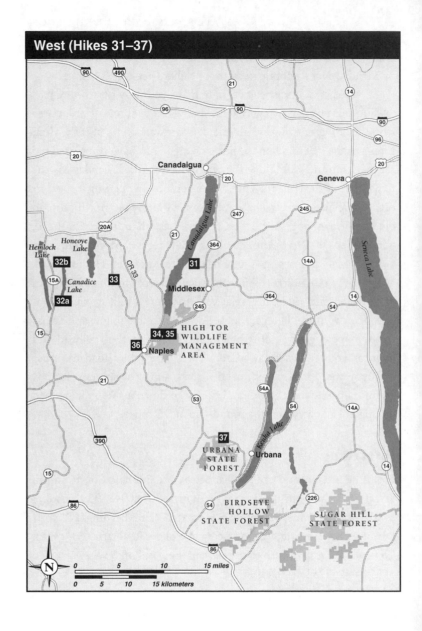

West (Hikes 31–37)

West

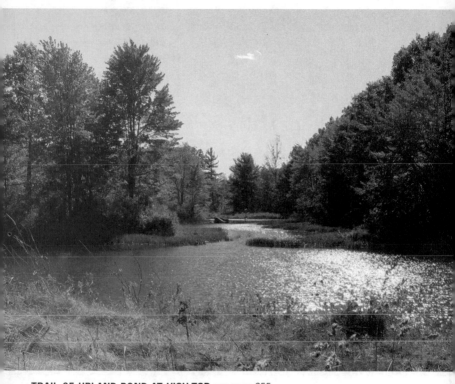

TRAIL 35 UPLAND POND AT HIGH TOR *see page 255*

Bare Hill Unique Area

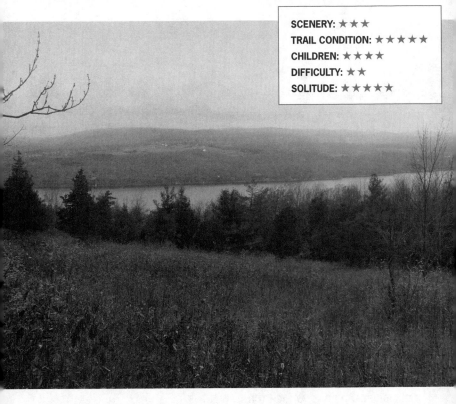

SCENERY: ★ ★ ★
TRAIL CONDITION: ★ ★ ★ ★ ★
CHILDREN: ★ ★ ★ ★
DIFFICULTY: ★ ★
SOLITUDE: ★ ★ ★ ★ ★

GPS TRAILHEAD COORDINATES: N42° 44.806'   W77° 18.159'

DISTANCE & CONFIGURATION: Upper Trail, 1.6-mile out-and-back; Lower Trail, 1.4-mile out-and-back; 3.0 miles total

HIKING TIME: 1.5 hours

HIGHLIGHTS: Scenic vista

ELEVATION: 1,370' at trailhead; 1,528' at Council Rock

ACCESS: Open 24/7; no fees or permits required

MAPS: DEC Bare Hill Unique Area map: **dec.ny.gov/lands/38798.html**

FACILITIES: None

WHEELCHAIR ACCESS: No

COMMENTS: The area consists of two out-and-back trips approximately 1.5 miles each. By combining them, you could extend your trip to 3 miles.

CONTACTS: NYSDEC Region 8 Headquarters, 585-226-2466, **dec.ny.gov/lands/37438.html**

Overview

In a region of forested hills, the aptly named Bare Hill is wrought with rumors about the origin of its unique character. Regardless of the veracity of the legends surrounding the hill, the trail here offers pleasant out-in-the-open hiking, as well as some scenic vistas of Canandaigua Lake.

Route Details

According to one local legend, the hill—known as Ge-nun-de-wah in the Seneca language—is the location of a myth about how Bare Hill became "bare." The paraphrased story goes like this: While out canoe-ing, a young Seneca boy found a multicolored snake and brought it back to his village. The boy fed his pet snake insects, frogs, and small mammals, but the snake's appetite was insatiable, and it soon required ever-larger prey and the assistance of fellow villagers to acquire the quantity needed. Food became increasingly scarce, and the predator grew to such immense size that its body soon encompassed the entire village, eventually devouring all within, with the exception of a brother and sister. In a dream, the boy saw the one vulnerable spot to shoot the snake with a poison arrow. The boy attempted to kill the snake, which did not die when shot but rather thrashed severely while rolling down the hill and destroying tree and bush alike, leaving the hill bare. According to some, from that point forward the hill held special meaning for the Seneca Indians and was the location for great councils and special rites. It's an interesting and compelling story, but some say it is utterly false. Peter Jemison, the author of the Department of Environmental Conservation unit man-agement plan's history section, states that no Seneca elder has given any credence to the story. In fact, one elder went so far as to call it "a white man's tale." The true origin of the story—as well as its veracity, meaning, or place in history—is beyond the scope of this book, but suffice it to say that the legend is now tied to the area.

Bare Hill Unique Area

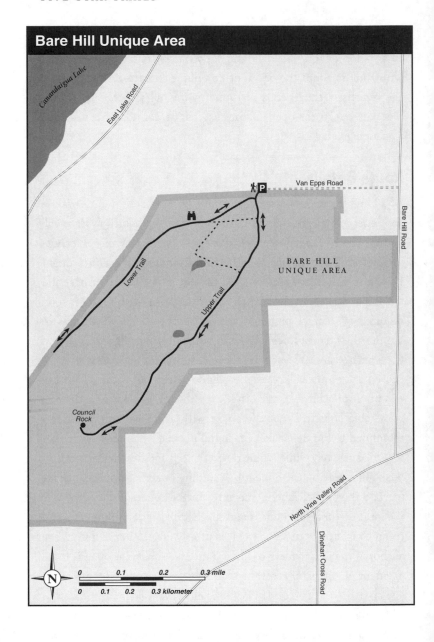

Two trails explore the Bare Hill Unique Area: an Upper Trail and Lower Trail. The Lower Trail, just shy of 0.75 mile to the end, follows an old access road and dips down from the open fields near the trailhead into a dense hardwood forest below. Although a perfectly pleasant walk, the trail simply ends in the middle of the forest and offers little in the way of views or sense of accomplishment at its conclusion. That's a shame because connecting the Upper and Lower Trails would create a very sensible and pleasant loop. In autumn, after the leaves have fallen, or during the winter, glimpses of Canandaigua Lake may be visible on your return trip, but that view would be completely obstructed when the trees are leafed out. However, some of the best vistas of Canandaigua Lake are available less than a third of the way along this trail. To take in these views, bear right at the kiosk and continue southwest less than 0.25 mile. Around this point, you will reach a fork in the trail where a short access road continues to the left, while the Lower Trail continues to descend to the right. This area has a broad sloping field to the west that allows you to take in a commanding view of the southern tip of Canandaigua Lake. You can continue along the Lower Trail to its terminus a little more than 0.5 mile ahead and return, or head back to the kiosk and begin the Upper Trail.

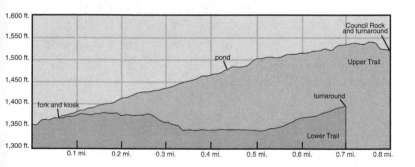

The trail to Council Rock, the Upper Trail, is the real gem here and—unless the two trails can be connected via some future loop—is my recommended hike (though you should also head to the scenic vista mentioned earlier). Bear left at the kiosk, and follow the old access road south. The trail is unmarked but is mowed, so it is easy to follow. The trail climbs nearly the entire way to Council Rock, but the grade is very easy, climbing 150 feet over the next 0.8 mile. Most trails in Central New York and the Finger Lakes that follow drumlin hilltops are covered in hardwood forest. Though their shade is a welcome reprieve during the height of summer, the forest often obscures views of the surrounding valleys and hilltops. Not so at the Bare Hill Unique Area. The hilltop is mostly open fields dotted with small evergreens, a very different hilltop environment and habitat than found throughout the region. As you climb you will catch glimpses of these valleys to the east but not of Canandaigua Lake to the west; a band of evergreens and the typical hardwood forest grow downslope and are just high enough to obscure the lake. About 0.25 mile along this trail, you encounter a road leading off to your right. When I visited, I mistook this road as a connector to the Lower Trail, but in fact it leads to the first of two ponds found in the area. You pass the second of these ponds in another 0.25 mile, at a little less than 0.5 mile total. Clearly man-made, these reservoirs provide an important water resource to upland wildlife and perhaps are a leading reason the area is popular with hunters in the fall. Just before reaching Council Rock you will pass over a small knoll before descending to the bonfire area. Atop this knoll are the only views of the lake along this section of trail. As the surrounding forest continues to grow taller, it won't be long before this vista is obscured as well. Continue down to Council Rock to reach the end of the trip, approximately 0.8 mile. Return the way you came for a total length of 1.6 miles.

Nearby Attractions

Though technically not an attraction, the area at Council Rock is where a bonfire is lit as part of the annual Ring of Fire festival along

Canandaigua Lake. The fire is lit on the Saturday before Labor Day. Lakeside fires and flares are also ignited to create a ring of fire around the lake. The tradition is rumored to have started as a Seneca ritual giving thanks for a bountiful harvest by lighting cattails along the lakeshore. Honeoye and Keuka Lakes also celebrate the tradition, and though I have not had the opportunity to see the spectacle, pictures from the event are truly impressive.

Directions

From the north: From NY 5/US 20/Eastern Boulevard in Canandaigua, head south on NY 384 South/East Lake Road. Follow it south 8.2 miles, and turn right onto Town Line Road. Take the first left onto Bare Hill Road, at 1.1 miles. Turn right onto Van Epps Road at 1 mile. Continue 0.3 mile to the end of the road, where you'll find parking.

From the south: From I-390, take Exit 2 (NY 415/Cohocton/Naples). Turn right on Cohocton Loon Lake Road/CR 121. Turn right onto Maple Avenue/NY 415, at 0.4 mile. Turn left onto NY 371 North/North Main Street, at 0.6 mile. Follow NY 371 north 4.8 miles and continue straight on NY 21 North/Naples Street for 6.0 miles. Turn right onto NY 245 North. Turn left on NY 364, at 8.8 miles. Turn right after 0.4 mile, and continue on NY 364 North. Turn left onto CR 10/North Vine Valley Road at 2.2 miles. Take the first right onto Bare Hill Road at 0.9 mile. Take the first left onto Van Epps Road, at 0.7 mile, and continue 0.3 mile to the end of the road, where you'll find parking.

SCENERY: ★ ★ ★
TRAIL CONDITION: ★ ★ ★ ★ ★
CHILDREN: ★ ★ ★ ★
DIFFICULTY: ★
SOLITUDE: ★ ★ ★ ★ ★

GPS TRAILHEAD COORDINATES: (south trailhead) N42° 41.5065'   W77° 34.1436'
(north trailhead) N42° 44.6179'   W77° 34.4207'

DISTANCE & CONFIGURATION: 8.0-mile out-and-back

HIKING TIME: 2–3 hours

HIGHLIGHTS: Pristine lake, old foundations

ELEVATION: 1,125' at trailhead, with no significant rise

ACCESS: Open 24/7; no fees or permits required

MAPS: hemlockandcanadicelakes.com/hcl_hiking_0_index.htm; DEC Hemlock-Canadice
State Forest brochure: **dec.ny.gov/lands/66521.html**

FACILITIES: None

WHEELCHAIR ACCESS: No

COMMENTS: Canadice Lake is one of two lakes that provide Rochester with its drinking
water. Thus special conditions apply to preserve water quality. A list of these restrictions is
available at **dec.ny.gov/regs/13943.html.** Most of these regulations regard boating, fishing,
and camping, but hikers should be aware that swimming for both people and pets is strictly
prohibited. Dogs are permitted here on leash or under control at all times.

CONTACTS: NYSDEC State Land Management, 607-776-2165, **dec.ny.gov/lands
/66521.html**

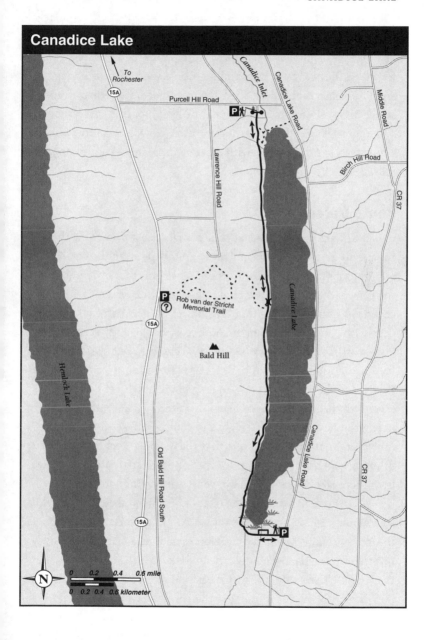

Canadice Lake

To Rochester

15A

Purcell Hill Road

Canadice Inlet

Canadice Lake Road

Middle Road

Birch Hill Road

Lawrence Hill Road

P

CR 37

P
?

Rob van der Stricht
Memorial Trail

15A

Canadice Lake

Bald Hill

Hemlock Lake

Old Bald Hill Road South

Canadice Lake Road

CR 37

15A

P

N

0   0.2   0.4   0.6 mile

0   0.2 0.4 0.6 kilometer

Overview

The hike along Canadice Lake's western shore follows access roads for the Rochester Water Department. Consequently the trail is broad and in excellent condition. Slightly more invigorating than the lake strolls found elsewhere in the book, the length of this trail results in a bit more solitude than the shorter, often-crowded lake trails. Total trip length is 8 miles, but with clear footing and level terrain, the mileage flies by.

Route Details

Canadice Lake is the smallest and perhaps least known of the 11 commonly recognized Finger Lakes. There are a number of "12th" and "thumb" lakes, but most of these other finger lakes do not share the common attributes of a true finger lake. The generally accepted criteria of a finger lake are that the body of water is narrow, long, and deep with a more or less north-south axis. Geologically speaking the Finger Lakes were formed when river valleys were deeply scoured and dammed during the Pleistocene ice age. Three miles long, Canadice Lake is the shortest finger lake in length, but at 91 feet deep it ranks seventh in depth. Hemlock Lake, Canadice's neighbor, ranks eighth in length (7 miles long) and eighth in depth (90 feet). The two lakes' other common characteristic is that they supply Rochester with its drinking water, which in turn leads to another attribute that makes both these lakes a desirable hiking destination: They are wild lakes.

For more than a century, Rochester has been acquiring the land surrounding Hemlock and Canadice Lakes to preserve the quality of the city's drinking water supply. Homesteads and farms have slowly reverted to forestland, and now the two lakes are the only finger lakes that could be properly categorized as undeveloped. Without camps, homes, and private land dotting the shore, hikers have unfettered access to these uniquely wild shores. Both lakes have trails along their shores, but only Canadice has a continuous trail from end to end (see Nearby Attractions for more about Hemlock Lake trails).

Bear in mind that although Canadice and Hemlock Lakes are within state forests, there are more restrictive regulations in place, most related to fishing and boating, but a few pertaining specifically to hikers. First, camping is prohibited throughout the property. Second, swimming, bathing, or otherwise coming into contact with water is not only prohibited but against the law. Be mindful that the same prohibition about water contact applies to pets. For a full list of regulations, see the state lands brochure available on the Department of Environmental Conservation website or the complete list of regulations at **dec.ny.gov/regs/13943.html.**

The trail description and mileage are based on the southern access point, but hikers might want to consider using the northern parking area, especially in winter when roadside parking in the south might be plowed in or buried with snowbanks.

Head eastward, past the vehicle barrier gate, along the gravel access road. A wetland sprawls to either side of the road, and glimpses of Canadice Lake can be caught to the north through the surrounding trees. About 0.25 mile in, the road passes by a bench near an opening in the wetland vegetation to the north, where the first real vistas of the lake are available. A little farther ahead, the road swings northward and the trail passes within feet of the lake. As you make your way northward, the trail climbs slightly higher above the lakeshore and eventually travels farther away. Other than the beautifully pristine and wild shores of Canadice Lake, there is little to note along the service road, with perhaps two exceptions.

The first items of note are the remains of old homesteads dotted along the trail to either side. Foundations, cellar holes, and fireplaces are all that remain of the settlements and houses that once lined these shores. The service road and the crumbling masonry are the only sights to break the illusion of walking beside an untouched lake. Most of the foundations can be seen along the southern half of the lake and virtually disappear from view as the road shifts slightly away from the lakeshore and heads farther north.

The only other notable feature encountered along the trail is a wooden footbridge at 2.25 miles. On some old maps this footbridge is located near Rob's Trail, a 1.75-mile loop/access trail that runs through Nature Conservancy property up to Old Bald Hill Road South/NY 15A. The trail was built in 2008 and connects Canadice and Hemlock Lakes. The connection to the Nature Conservancy property is a steep ascent, but once on conservancy land the trail is level. This could be a nice diversion with some added difficulty, but I did not make the trip when I visited.

The service road continues another 1.75 miles to the northern parking area, but you could just as easily turn around when you see the sprawling field and dam at the northern end of the lake, just shy of 4 miles. Beyond, there is little else to see than the parking area, but you still have all the great views of the wild lake on your 4-mile return to the southern parking area.

Nearby Attractions

Hemlock Lake also has trails along its shore, though I did not visit them and can't attest to their quality. An old road once followed its eastern shore, and there is an idea to use this old road to connect the northern and southern trails. Trail maps and directions to the trailhead are available at the sites listed previously for Canadice Lake. The optimist in me hopes that someday both lakes are encircled with trails and fully connected by Rob's Trail for an ideal finger lake figure eight.

Directions

From the intersection of NY 21 and US 20 in Canandaigua, head west on NY 5/US 20/Buffalo Road for 2.2 miles. Turn left on NY 64/US 20A and follow it 4.2 miles south. Turn left to stay on US 20A. Continue southwest for 7.9 miles, and turn left on CR 37. At 3.7 miles, turn right to stay on CR 37. Follow it 4.8 miles, and turn right on Johnson Hill Road. Turn right on Canadice Lake Road after 0.4 mile, and follow it north 1.2 miles to the large pulloff on the west side of the road, just past the vehicle barrier gate and trailhead.

Wesley Hill
Nature Preserve

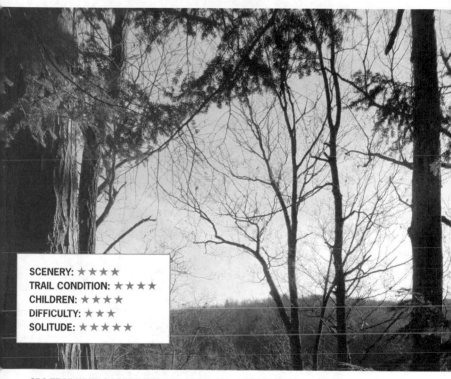

SCENERY: ★ ★ ★ ★
TRAIL CONDITION: ★ ★ ★ ★
CHILDREN: ★ ★ ★ ★
DIFFICULTY: ★ ★
SOLITUDE: ★ ★ ★ ★ ★

GPS TRAILHEAD COORDINATES: N42° 43.452'   W77° 28.069'

DISTANCE & CONFIGURATION: 4.1-mile loop

HIKING TIME: 1.5–2.5 hours

HIGHLIGHTS: Pond, meandering streams, isolated glens, secluded gorge

ELEVATION: 1,790' at trailhead; 1,400' at lowest point along trail

ACCESS: Daily, sunrise–sunset; no fees or permits required

MAPS: fllt.org (search for "Wesley Hill")

FACILITIES: None

WHEELCHAIR ACCESS: No

COMMENTS: Sections of the trail network by the Wesley Road entrance are closed during bow hunting season. Those sections are not described here but can be added for an extended trip.

CONTACTS: Finger Lakes Land Trust, 607-275-9487, **fllt.org/protected_lands /protected_lands1.php?id=31**

Wesley Hill Nature Preserve

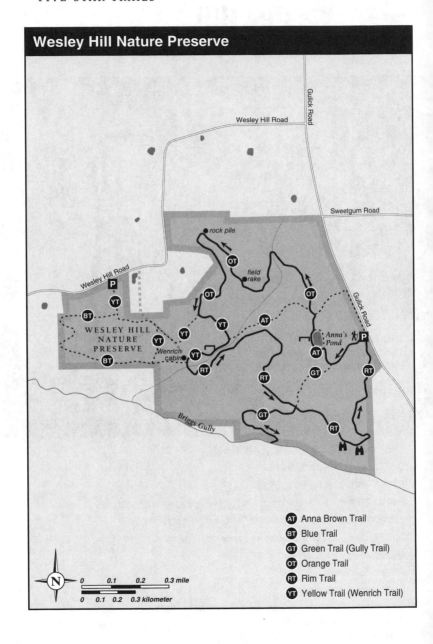

AT Anna Brown Trail
BT Blue Trail
GT Green Trail (Gully Trail)
OT Orange Trail
RT Rim Trail
YT Yellow Trail (Wenrich Trail)

Overview

Packed into the 390-acre preserve is a wide variety of hiking environs. With abandoned orchards, open fields, successional forests, stony streams, and deep gullies, you'll find a little bit of everything you expect from a Finger Lakes trail. Because it lies slightly off the beaten path in this region, you get a touch of privacy while experiencing all the Finger Lakes have to offer.

Route Details

The trail network at Wesley Hill Nature Preserve has many interconnected trails, so the options to increase or decrease your trip length are varied. I visited the preserve during hunting season, so the western section of the preserve past the Wenrich cabin—the Blue Trail and most of the Yellow Trail—was closed to hikers. I chose a route that took in most of the other sections and tried to hit all the highlights. Generally speaking, the red (Anna Brown and Rim) and Green Trails feature the streams and gullies, while the Orange Trail highlights the abandoned orchards and successional forests.

The trails begin on the southern end of the parking area, just past the information kiosk. Follow the Green/Red (Anna Brown) Trail a short way downhill to where the two diverge. The green Gully Trail continues straight, while the red Anna Brown Trail travels along the right

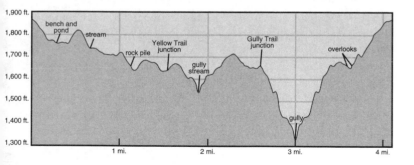

fork. Bear right and quickly reach another fork, just as Anna's Pond and an open field come into view. Both trails are sections along the Anna Brown Trail and reconnect north of the pond. The right-hand option follows the eastern side of the pond through the edge of the forest, while the left-hand option follows a mown path along a berm that circumnavigates the western edge of the pond. About midway along this mown path, you'll find a small bench to sit beside the pond and enjoy the peaceful setting. Where the two trails rejoin, continue northward and back into the forest.

As you reenter the forest, bear left and cross a seasonal stream. Once on the other bank, the trail intersects the start of the Orange Trail. The red Anna Brown Trail continues ahead along the northern rim of an ever-deepening gully to the Wenrich cabin, 0.25 mile from the Yellow Trail intersection. Here, the gully is the shallow stream that the trail just crossed, but farther ahead, where the northern trails rejoin the red Anna Brown Trail, it is far more dramatic. Meanwhile, turn right and follow the Orange Trail into the northern sections of the preserve. Originally just 90 acres in 1999, the Wesley Hill Nature Preserve has been expanded to 390 acres through purchases and gifts. The Orange Trail meanders through three of these tracts: the Anna Brown Tract, the White Tract, and the Alpaugh Tract. These tracts feature a mixture of forest types as old fields and orchards transition back into the forest.

The Orange Trail begins with a brief climb, follows the contours of the neighboring hill, and then descends to another stream crossing, where a field is slowly succeeding back into forest. Once across the stream, take a sharp left and continue south through the field briefly before the trail reenters the forest and then turns briefly west again. As the trail bends northward, it winds downhill a little more steeply as it approaches the northern edge of the preserve. Shortly after passing an old foundation (pile of stones) on the right, the trail switches back southward and follows the contour of the hill as it winds southward.

At 1.5 miles, you reach the intersection with the Wenrich Trail. The yellow-marked Wenrich Trail continues straight ahead as well as to the left. Ahead is the section that is closed during hunting season, while the curving path to the left connects with the red Anna Brown Trail in less than 0.25 mile. Turn left, pass through a small depression, and soon leave behind the oaks and maples and head into a hemlock forest. As the gully comes into sight, the Yellow Trail intersects the red Anna Brown Trail.

Turn right, westward, on the combined Red and Yellow Trails, and head downhill along the northern rim of the gully. Shortly after passing a small bench beside the trail, you veer away from the gully and can glimpse the Wenrich cabin, with its dark brown wood and light blue trim, to your right, at 1.9 miles. The cabin is closed, but on the porch are brochures, newsletters, and informative posters from the Finger Lakes Land Trust.

The Yellow Trail continues straight into the western section of the preserve, the Wenrich-Havens Tract. Unfortunately, when I visited, this section was closed for bow hunting season, but during other times of the year a combination of the yellow- and blue-marked trails could add another 1.25 miles to your excursion. If you do add this section to your trip, you will return to this point. To complete the loop, follow the red Rim Trail south and head down into the hemlock-lined gully. Slabs of shale and debris clutter the gully floor, and you will have to rock-hop across the narrow stream before beginning a steep ascent to the gully's opposing southern rim. Some interesting scenes and short cascades can be glimpsed down within the gully as you climb and traverse the southern rim for approximately 0.25 mile.

The trail eventually leads eastward away from the gully and enters into a predominantly oak hardwood forest. Shortly after, the trail bends more directly south and you cross several small seasonal tributaries of Briggs Gully. At 2.65 miles, you intersect the green-marked Gully Trail. On the left is a more direct route back to the parking area, about 0.3 mile to the north, while to your right is the steep descent to Briggs Gully. The Finger Lakes Land Trust owns only a portion of the property along the gully, but it is an interesting and wild scene worth the 200-foot descent and additional mile.

Heading down toward the gully, the trail descends immediately and grows ever steeper as you proceed. The trail initially follows a long westward-slanting cut across the steep hill. Approximately halfway along the descent, you make a short but steep scramble down a slippery slope, after which the trail turns eastward. The descent slackens a bit, and you'll cross by and over some deeply incised streamlets before turning sharply left for the final steep scramble. You will likely need your hands free along the last portion as you enter the wild gully below. It's clear why this is referred to as a gully rather than a gorge, since it's not nearly as deeply incised as other gorges in the region. Nevertheless, the spot is a perfect setting to stop and rest before beginning the return climb.

Once you return to the Rim Trail intersection, turn right and follow the Red Trail eastward. The trail crosses a couple of tributary streams and reaches a peninsula-like point in about 0.25 mile, at 3.66 miles overall. At two points there are obscured views across Briggs Gully to the opposing ridge. Though certainly not panoramic vistas, the views have an open feel, especially after the leaves have fallen.

After a sharp right turn, the trail swings nearly due north and begins the final section and climb—100 feet over the next 0.3 mile. There is a bench about midway along the climb back to the parking area along Gulick Road, in case you want to pause and rest.

Directions

From the intersection of NY 20A and East Lake Road in Honeoye, turn onto East Lake Road and head south 0.6 mile. Turn left onto CR 33/Pinewood Hill Road. Take the first right onto Pinewood Hill Road, after 0.4 mile. At 1.1 miles, bear right where Pinewood Hill Road becomes Gulick Road. Continue 3.3 miles to the parking area on the right.

Conklin Gully/ Parish Glen

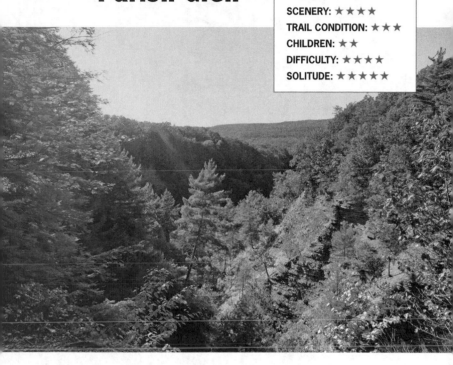

SCENERY: ★ ★ ★ ★
TRAIL CONDITION: ★ ★ ★
CHILDREN: ★ ★
DIFFICULTY: ★ ★ ★ ★
SOLITUDE: ★ ★ ★ ★ ★

GPS TRAILHEAD COORDINATES: N42° 38.110'   W77° 22.034'

DISTANCE & CONFIGURATION: 1.6-mile loop; longer trip available if combined with the High Tor loop.

HIKING TIME: 1 hour

HIGHLIGHTS: Waterfalls, scenic gorge, panoramic views

ELEVATION: 768' at trailhead; 1,157' at highest point along trail

ACCESS: Open 24/7; no fees or permits required

MAPS: Finger Lakes Trail Conference: Sheet B1

FACILITIES: None

WHEELCHAIR ACCESS: No

COMMENTS: Parts of the trail traverse the edge of a sheer cliff, so caution is advised. Because cliff edges are often undercut, approach cautiously and never tread where you are uncertain of your footing.

CONTACTS: NYSDEC Region 8 Headquarters, 585-226-2466, **dec.ny.gov/outdoor /24439.html**

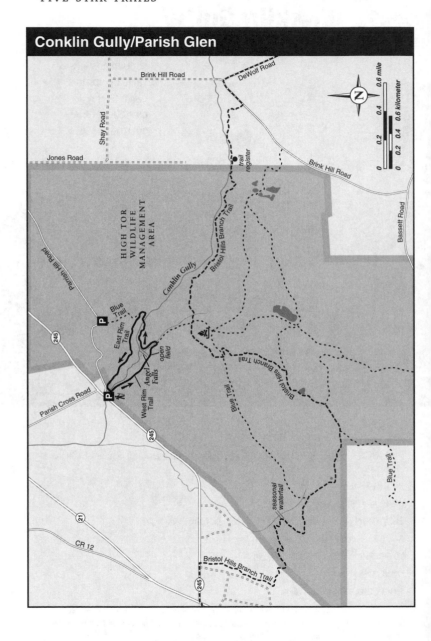

Conklin Gully/Parish Glen

Overview

Conklin Gully can be hiked as a short circuit or as the beginning and end of a much longer loop through the High Tor Wildlife Management Area. The short loop along the rim of a deeply incised ravine offers a short but steep climb with the quick reward of two steep waterfalls and some scenic vistas. The trail is mostly unmarked and, due to sheer cliffs, not a good choice for young children.

Route Details

Conklin Gully, also known as Parish Glen, can be explored in two different ways: either as a creek walk or as a rim circuit following the West and East Rim Trails. The creek walk involves a great deal of scrambling and sloshing through the creek bed. Be advised that it includes many sections of rock climbing over wet and slippery surfaces. The creek walk is very difficult; this often-described route includes climbing through the gorge and then up the steep gorge walls, so you can return along one of the rim trails; the rationale is that climbing through the gorge is so difficult that you would not want to try and go back down the same route. I don't recommend any route that does not include an option of turning back should you feel unable to continue. The inadvisability is compounded during

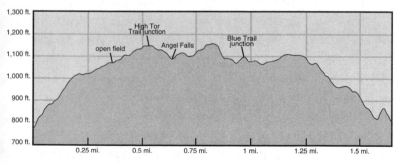

FIVE-STAR TRAILS

the spring and times of high water because sections could become impassable, and because returning can prove equally dangerous, hikers could find themselves in a dire predicament. Consequently, I don't advise hikers using this route to explore the glen. The better alternative is hiking along the rim trails, which are accessible during any season and are an equally scenic option. Should you choose the ill-advised option of exploring within the gorge, do so only in times of low water, never go alone, and do not begin climbing anything you would not feel comfortable climbing back down.

To take in the most dramatic vistas of the gully, I recommend a counterclockwise route: following the West Rim Trail and returning along the East Rim Trail. Additionally, if you choose to circumnavigate the gorge in the clockwise direction, by following the East Rim Trail and returning along the West Rim Trail, it can be hard to discern where to start. In the counterclockwise direction, the most difficult and least scenic part of the trip is at the beginning and leaves the vistas of the gorge for the middle and end of your trip.

West Rim Trail

To begin the trip, head to the eastern end of the parking area and look for an unmarked and worn path beside a small kiosk. Head south along this path and pass by a smaller worn path leading down to the stream on your left. This side path will likely be where you cross the stream when you return to the parking area. The main path becomes a worn road that continues uphill on the west side of the creek. The ascent is quite steep, close to 400 feet of elevation gain over roughly 0.5 mile. Along the climb you intersect a road coming in from your right. This road briefly leads away from the gorge but rejoins the main route about 0.1 mile farther ahead. Numerous paths on your left lead to the gorge's rim to provide glimpses into the gorge.

At 0.4 mile, the trail begins to level off and enters into an open field. You can skirt the edge of this field along footpaths closer to the gorge's rim or continue south through the clearing and reenter the forest. Shortly after entering the forest, you reach an intersection along the trail and the first trail markers. To your left, partially marked in blue, is the circuit around the gorge's rim. Straight ahead, also marked in blue, is the side trail that leads farther into the High Tor Wildlife Management Area (see page 255 for trail description). If you plan to add this trail to your trip, you will visit upper Conklin Gully, a much milder and more tranquil glen than the deeply incised ravine ahead. To complete the circuit, return along the East Rim Trail described below.

East Rim Trail

The trail heads east and dips down to cross one of the tributaries of Conklin Gully. When this stream reaches the gully, it cascades 120 feet into the deep ravine below. Unfortunately, this waterfall, often referred to as Angel Falls, is often dry and not always visible.

Once across the stream, the blue-marked trail turns to your left and heads north following the stream. The trail follows the southern rim of the gorge along a peninsula-like protrusion that juts out where the two streams that have carved the gorge meet. Shrouded in hemlocks, the tip of the protrusion is a dramatic scene with steep cliffs all around. However, the canopy is so dense that it's also eerily dark and photos often require a flash. As the trail swings southward, the canopy thins and light begins to filter back onto the trail. Far below to your left, a waterfall along the eastern tributary is framed by trees precariously clinging to the sheer gorge walls. Vistas and dramatic scenery abound, but, sadly, the obstructing trees make these scenes difficult to capture with a camera. Fortunately there is a broad opening a little ahead where a panorama and an excellent photo op of the steep cliffs and small waterfall await.

The trail soon begins a steep descent, and you will cross the stream that carves the gorge. This crossing is roughly 0.3 mile from the intersection of the High Tor Blue Trail, or roughly the halfway point for the rim loop. Once across, a worn footpath leads down into the gorge on your left, while the designated trail, still marked in blue, leads away from the stream and up a small hill. Follow the Blue Trail uphill and southeast. Shortly after, the trail swings northward and you reach the final trail intersection. To the right, the blue-marked trail continues downhill a little over 0.25 mile to an access point along Parrish Hill Road. Instead, take a left on an unmarked path that follows the eastern rim of the gorge. It begins as a worn path along a narrow ridge between the gorge on your left and a tiny gully on your right. The path is nearly as wide as the ridge, and within 0.25 mile you return to views of Conklin Gully. This side of the gorge is dotted with hardwoods, so dramatic views of the gorge are more likely in fall or winter. Nonetheless, the sheer cliffs are visible and accompany you as you scramble down nearly 400 feet over the next 0.4 mile. The trail is little more than a worn footpath with many steep gravelly sections. The easiest way to reach the parking area is to rock-hop across the stream for a 1.6-mile round-trip, or 9.2 miles if you included the High Tor loop.

Directions

From the north: From NY 5/US 20/Eastern Boulevard in Canandaigua, head south on NY 384 South/East Lake Road. Follow it south for 12.1 miles and turn left to stay on NY 384. At 0.4 mile, turn right on NY 245 South. Follow NY 245 South 7.2 miles; the parking area is on the left just after passing Parrish Hill Road and crossing Conklin Gully Creek.

  From the south: From I-390, take Exit 2 (NY 415/Cohocton/Naples). Turn right on Cohocton Loon Lake Road/CR 121. Turn right onto Maple Avenue/NY 415, at 0.4 mile. Turn left onto NY 371 North/North Main Street, at 0.6 mile. Follow NY 371 north 4.8 miles and continue straight on NY 21 North/Naples Street for 6.0 miles. Turn right onto NY 245 North. Follow it 1.7 miles, and the parking area will be on the right, just before Parrish Hill Road.

High Tor Wildlife Management Area

35

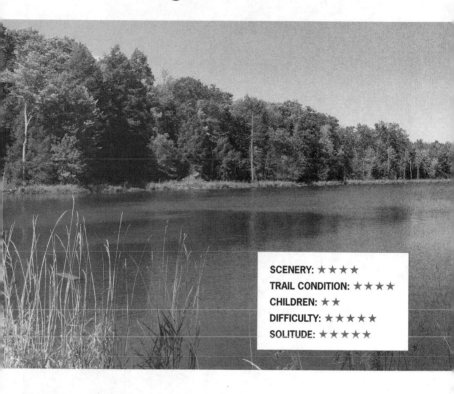

SCENERY: ★ ★ ★ ★
TRAIL CONDITION: ★ ★ ★ ★
CHILDREN: ★ ★
DIFFICULTY: ★ ★ ★ ★ ★
SOLITUDE: ★ ★ ★ ★ ★

GPS TRAILHEAD COORDINATES: N42° 38.110'   W77° 22.034'

DISTANCE & CONFIGURATION: 9.2-mile loop

HIKING TIME: 4–5 hours

HIGHLIGHTS: Secluded woodland, scenic vista, open fields, isolated ponds, glens

ELEVATION: 743' at trailhead; 1,836' at highest point along trail

ACCESS: Open 24/7; no fees or permits required

MAPS: Finger Lakes Trail Conference: Sheet B1

FACILITIES: None

WHEELCHAIR ACCESS: No

COMMENTS: Sections of this hike are near sheer vertical cliffs. Be careful when approaching undercut cliffs.

CONTACTS: NYSDEC Region 8 Headquarters, 585-226-2466, **dec.ny.gov/outdoor /24439.html**

High Tor Wildlife Management Area

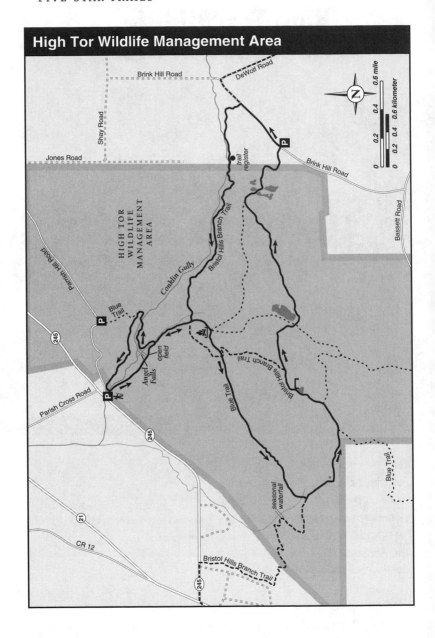

Overview

The High Tor Wildlife Management Area is made up of three sections that total 6,100 acres. The trail described here circumnavigates the larger of these sections (3,400 acres). The 9.2-mile loop has a myriad of interwoven trails and access roads, so there are options to either lengthen or shorten your trip. The route below encompasses/bisects many of these options and highlights the various habitats and ecosystems found across this upland plateau.

Route Details

Several parking areas provide access to the High Tor Wildlife Management Area. The route I chose starts and ends with the Conklin Gully rim loop, but it also passes by or intersects most of the alternative access points. If you choose to start at one of the alternate parking areas, I've divided the trail into different segments noting the total miles along each section to simplify your trip planning.

Lower Conklin Gully

(west side; 0.5 mile to beginning of Side Trail; 1 mile to campsite 2)
The first portion of the trail is described in the Conklin Gully/Parish Glen hike, page 252, and includes a 400-foot climb over roughly 0.5 mile. When you reach the intersection with the blue-marked trail,

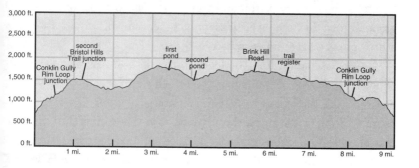

continue to climb south. From the intersection the trail climbs another 400 feet over the next 0.5 mile, for a total of roughly 800 feet of elevation gain in roughly 1 mile. Approximately 0.3 mile from the Conklin Gully loop described here, you intersect Bristol Hills Trail, marked in orange. You first pass the westward continuation of this trail on your right, and then shortly after you pass the section that traverses the upper Conklin Gully on your left. Should you choose to follow the entire loop, this is the point to which you will return before completing the lower Conklin Gully portion of the trail. Meanwhile, continue straight ahead and climb for the next 0.25 mile. At the conclusion of the climb, you reach an open grassy area and the next portion of the trip.

Side Trail *(1.4 miles)*

When you reach the clearing, bear right toward the fire pit. A swath of trees is cut along the hillside here, providing a wide vista of Canandaigua Lake to the north. The canopy of the forest downhill obstructs this view, but if you stand on the fire-pit ledge, you gain enough elevation to take in the lake. As the forest downslope grows, this vantage might be lost, but during the winter and fall the scene is even more panoramic. The clearing and facilities (campsite 2) are part of a network of campsites available in the High Tor Wildlife Management Area. However, camping at these sites is reserved for organized groups such as the Boy Scouts. Camping is by permit and only in designated areas for these groups during the hunting off-season. All other camping activities are strictly prohibited within the preserve.

Continue south past the log lean-to and bear-resistant food storage on your right. At this point you reach an intersection of several roads. To the left, east, is the main access road for this camping area. Straight ahead is a short bypass road that connects to the Bristol Hills Connection and Upland Ponds sections described later. To the right, with barely discernible blue marks, is the Bristol Hills Side Trail. Turn right and follow the blue-marked road southwest. Blue trail markers are found on trees to either side of this road, but dense brush often obscures the paints. The broad grassy road cuts a wide swath through the hilltop forest and gradually descends a little over 200 feet for just shy of 1 mile. Less than 0.25 mile along this road, you re-intersect the orange-marked Bristol Hills Trail. This is the return point should you choose to bypass the Upland Ponds and upper Conklin Gully trails. Continue straight roughly 0.75 mile to where the road concludes and the Side Trail heads slightly uphill and into the surrounding forest. The trail begins a gentle climb over the next 0.5 mile. Shortly after entering into a hemlock grove and following the edge of a gully, the trail dips down into the gully and crosses its shallow stream. This stream eventually connects with the Conklin Gully stream and has cut its own less dramatic gully that parallels the Bristol Hills Trail, which you reconnect with once you reach the other side of the stream. At this junction you have a choice to follow the Bristol Hills Trail downhill and west to a seasonal waterfall, 0.5 mile, or to turn left, southeast, and continue the circuit. The side trip to the falls will add 1 mile to your total trip as well as 300 feet of descent and ascent. The falls and gully are handsome additions to the trip, but if the stream you crossed was dry, then the falls will also be dry and likely not worth the visit. Those looking for alternate access to High Tor should note that 1.1 miles northwest from this junction along the Bristol Hills Trail is an alternative access point along NY 245 in Naples, 0.6 mile past the waterfall.

Side Trail/Bristol Hills Connection *(0.6 mile to Side Trail departure; 1.25 miles to Upland Pond Road)*

Turn left, southeast, and immediately begin a steep climb of 400 feet over the next 0.5 mile. The trail is marked with both orange and blue paints. Roughly three-quarters of the way along this climb you pass a small pothole pond to the left of the trail. The climb ends at 0.6 mile, 3 miles overall, when you reach a T in the trail. To your right the blue-marked Side Trail continues 1.5 miles to another access point along East Hill Road. Turn left and follow the orange Bristol Hills Trail northeast. The next 0.3 mile is a fairly level trek along a broad

road to the first of the upland ponds along the trail. At the north end of this pond is a bench that makes an excellent stopping point, 3.4 miles from the start. A separate road winds around the north end of the pond and leads to another camping area (campsite 1). However, the Bristol Hills Trail continues to the left of the bench. The trail soon swings to your right and downhill and intersects a couple of roads, at 3.6 miles overall.

To the right is a road that passes by campsite 1 on its way 1.25 miles south to another access point along Bassett Road. To the left is the continuation of the Bristol Hills Trail, which, roughly 0.5 mile farther north, reconnects with the Side Trail described earlier. The route to explore the Upland Ponds section of the loop lies straight ahead.

Upland Ponds Roads *(2 miles to Brink Hill Road; 0.4 mile along Brink Hill Road to intersection with Upper Conklin Gully)*

I have assigned the name Upland Ponds Roads to the network of unmarked roads that thread through the eastern section of the management area. The roads are easy to follow and feature long sections of hiking out in the open and past several picturesque ponds. The first unmarked road, straight ahead at the four-way intersection, continues downhill and generally east about 0.25 mile before it swings southward and begins a slightly steeper decline. The second and much larger upland pond begins to come into view around this point, and the trail dips down into a marshy area near its southern outlet. A short way ahead, the top of a small berm is an excellent spot to snap some pictures of the pond. You can reach the berm along a worn path just past where the trail swings northeast again. Past the pond, the trail begins another climb, though now you are out in the open with forest flanking either side. Around 4.7 miles, you connect with another road that comes in from your right, or the south. This road meanders generally southeast to the access point along Bassett Road. Bear left, northeast, and head downhill about 0.25 mile to where the trail forks into yet another main access road. To your left the road continues about a mile back to campsite 2. Turn right and follow this road into another clearing where several ponds flank the trail to either side, at just over 5 miles overall. The ponds to the north are visible from the trail, but you will have to climb a short berm to see the ponds on the right. Past the ponds, the trail reenters the forest and begins a winding route roughly 0.3 mile to Brink Hill Road. Located along the east side of the road is yet another access point and large gravel parking area. Turn left and follow Brink Hill Road 0.4 mile to where it intersects the Bristol Hills Trail and another access point.

Upper Conklin Gully/Bristol Hills Trail
(1.8 miles to intersection with Side Trail)
Turn left off of Brink Hill Road and begin hiking west along the upper Conklin Gully portion of the Bristol Hills Trail. The narrow footpath meanders through small hardwoods about 0.3 mile before reaching the beginning of the gully. From this point forward you head mostly downhill and follow along the southern rim of an ever-deepening gully. Hemlocks soon dominate the trail, and you reach a trail register about 0.5 mile from the road, at just shy of 6.5 miles overall. The trail weaves away and back to the gully's edge multiple times. The gorge becomes progressively deeper, with its steep banks beside the trail growing ever steeper and more rugged as you travel farther west. After crossing a pair of short bridges, you'll come upon a vantage point on your right from which to view the now deeply cut gorge. Obscured by hemlocks, the view is interesting but a far cry from the spectacular vistas of the gorge along the Conklin Gully loop farther along. Past this view, the trail leads away from the gorge, and soon after dipping down and crossing a seasonal stream, it reconnects with the Side Trail at 1.8 miles from Brink Hill Road, or 7.8 miles overall.

Eastern Conklin Gully *(0.3 mile to reconnect with Conklin Gully Trail, 1.1 miles to return to parking area along NY 245)*
When you reconnect with the broad road, turn right and retrace your path back to the Conklin Gully rim loop. Since much of the spectacle of that gorge was absent along your ascent, I highly recommend that

you return along the eastern portion of the rim trail to take in all the scenic vistas. The return leg is described in the East Rim Trail section of the Conklin Gully/Parish Glen hike on page 253.

Directions

From the north: From NY 5/US 20/Eastern Boulevard in Canandaigua, head south on NY 384 South/East Lake Road. Follow it south 12.1 miles, and turn left to stay on NY 384. At 0.4 mile, turn right on NY 245 South. Follow NY 245 South for 7.2 miles; the parking area is on the left just after passing Parrish Hill Road and crossing Conklin Gully Creek.

From the south: From I-390, take Exit 2 (NY 415/Cohocton/ Naples). Turn right on Cohocton Loon Lake Road/CR 121. Turn right onto Maple Avenue/NY 415, at 0.4 mile. Turn left onto NY 371 North/North Main Street, at 0.6 mile. Follow NY 371 north 4.8 miles and continue straight on NY 21 North/Naples Street for 6.0 miles. Turn right onto NY 245 North. Follow it 1.7 miles, and the parking area will be on the right, just before Parrish Hill Road.

36 Grimes Glen

SCENERY: ★ ★ ★ ★ ★
TRAIL CONDITION: ★
CHILDREN: ★ ★ ★ ★
DIFFICULTY: ★
SOLITUDE: ★ ★ ★ ★

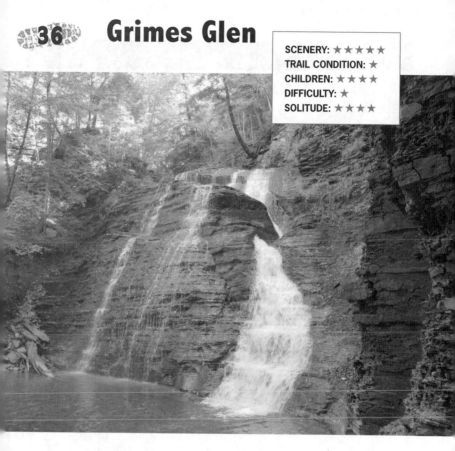

GPS TRAILHEAD COORDINATES: N42° 36.920'   W77° 24.821'

DISTANCE & CONFIGURATION: 1.0-mile out-and-back

HIKING TIME: 30 minutes–1 hour

HIGHLIGHTS: Two 60-foot waterfalls, creek walk, scenic gorge

ELEVATION: 835' at trailhead, with no significant rise

ACCESS: Daily, sunrise–sunset; no fees or permits required

MAPS: Finger Lakes Land Trust: **fllt.org** (search for "Grimes Glen"); Ontario County Parks Grimes Glen Brochure: **co.ontario.ny.us** (search for "Grimes Glen")

FACILITIES: Picnic tables

WHEELCHAIR ACCESS: No

COMMENTS: This trail is a creek walk, so expect to get your feet wet. Caution is always advised around slippery rocks.

CONTACTS: Ontario County of Public Works, 315-396-4000, **co.ontario.ny.us** (search for "Grimes Glen"); Friends of Grimes Glen, 585-374-2111

Grimes Glen

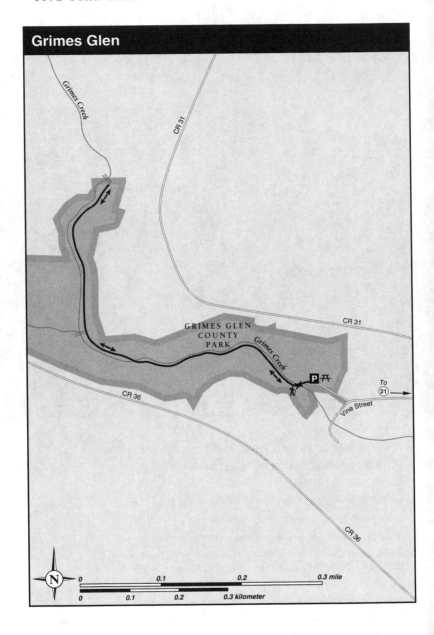

GRIMES GLEN
COUNTY
PARK

Grimes Creek

Grimes Creek

CR 31

CR 31

CR 36

CR 36

Vine Street

To
21

N

| 0 | | 0.1 | | 0.2 | | 0.3 mile |
| 0 | 0.1 | 0.2 | 0.3 kilometer | | | |

Overview

Though this is the shortest hike featured in the book, it is far from short on adventure. There is no actual trail of which to speak; rather you explore the glen along the creek bank or rock-hop through the creek itself. Splashing through the creek is often the easiest path, so expect to get your feet wet while admiring the gorge and the two 60-foot-high waterfalls. During times of high water—during the spring and after heavy rains—the creek may not be navigable or safe, so plan your trip accordingly.

Route Details

There is no real trail to describe here—hence the low trail condition rating—but do not let that deter you from exploring this pristine gem. Indeed, finding your route and getting your feet wet is half the fun in exploring this gorge, and I expect this will be the highlight for children and the young at heart. From the parking area, follow the road on your left past the picnic area, toward the bridge crossing Grimes Creek. A new bridge was installed in November 2012 and marks the beginning of the trail. Once across the bridge, you will find worn paths that weave along the south side of the creek. These footpaths continue eastward roughly 0.25 mile, where you encounter the first of the two 60-foot-tall waterfalls. At this point, the footpaths essentially disappear as the gorge narrows, but chances are that you will have already wandered out into the creek to snap some pictures of this beautiful waterfall. The broad waterfall, succinctly referred to as "first" falls, tumbles down to feed the creek and is more akin to a shower than the gushing flume that awaits you upstream.

From first falls onward, the gorge narrows, the shale bluffs become steeper, and you will have to make much of your way in the creek bed itself. The tumbling sounds of the falls, the babbling creek, and the wild nature of the gorge make it hard to believe that mere minutes earlier you were in the middle of the town of Naples. As you near "second" falls, you will most likely find yourself on the right-hand side of the creek. You come around a bend in the creek and enter into a 200-foot-tall shale-lined enclosure that surrounds the pool at the base of the falls. The falls bifurcate somewhere just out of view into a broad tumbling cascade on the left and a surging flume on the right. This flume is not fully visible when you first come upon the falls, but a small, slightly submerged ledge continues on the right and leads to a more desirable view of the falls. Indeed, a small cave cut into the shale wall at the end of this submerged ledge practically begs you to investigate. The pool at the base of the falls is only a couple of feet deep, so swimming is not really an option, but the setting alone is enough to offer a refreshing cool-down on a hot summer day.

Aside from the scenery, visitors might be interested to know that in 1882 a local geologist, D. Dana Luther, found a 350 million-year-old tree fossil in the glen. This partial fossil, commonly known as the Naples tree, is now housed at the New York State Museum in Albany and is considered one of the best examples of the earliest trees. The ancient tree was believed to be 15 feet tall and 1 foot in diameter. This tree had a leafy top but no branches and would likely not be recognizable as a tree to us today. In fact the Naples tree has more in common with the club mosses found throughout the region than it does with present-day trees. (See Connecticut Hill Wildlife Management Area: Bob Cameron Loop, on page 189, for a description of club mosses.) Bear in mind that this ancient tree existed during the Devonian period, when life was just beginning to leave the oceans and colonize the land. Indeed, the layers of shale that form the gorge walls are riddled with fossils from this prehistoric era, as is much of the shale found throughout Central New York; finding these fossils provides another attraction here. As is the case with other public lands, please leave fossils behind for future visitors. It is not only a courtesy for future generations but also against the law to remove plants, animals, rocks, or fossils from public lands and an essential part of the Leave No Trace ethic. This park's unique place in history and its obviously spectacular natural features are some of the reasons the land was acquired by the Finger Lakes Land Trust in 2008. Subsequently, the land was

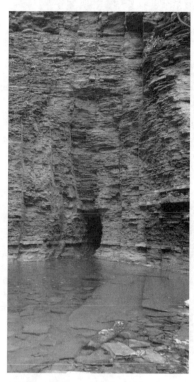

SMALL CAVE IN SHALE WALL

donated to Ontario County to handle maintenance of the park, but the land trust maintains a conservation easement that ensures the wild character of the park will continue—yet another successful example of a conservation and public works partnership for the enjoyment of all.

Directions

From the north: From NY 5/US 20/Eastern Boulevard in Canandaigua, head south on NY 384 South/East Lake Road. Follow it south for 12.1 miles, and turn left to stay on NY 384. At 0.4 mile, turn right onto NY 245 South. Follow it 8.8 miles and turn right on NY 21/North Main Street. Continue south through Naples for 1 mile, and turn left on Vine Street. Follow Vine Street 0.5 mile to its end. The parking area is just past a barrier gate, and ample parking is available past the brown building on your right.

From the south: From I-390, take Exit 2 (NY 415/Cohocton/Naples). Turn right on Cohocton Loon Lake Road/CR 121. Turn right onto Maple Avenue/NY 415, at 0.4 mile. Turn left onto NY 371 North/North Main Street, at 0.6 mile. Follow NY 371 north 4.8 miles and continue straight on NY 21 North/Naples Street. Turn left onto NY 21/South Main Street after 4.5 miles. Turn left on Vine Street at 0.5 mile, and follow directions above.

Urbana State Forest: Huckleberry Bog

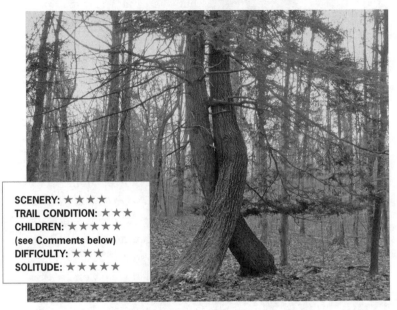

SCENERY: ★ ★ ★ ★
TRAIL CONDITION: ★ ★ ★
CHILDREN: ★ ★ ★ ★ ★
(see Comments below)
DIFFICULTY: ★ ★ ★
SOLITUDE: ★ ★ ★ ★ ★

GPS TRAILHEAD COORDINATES: N42° 28.669' W77° 14.525'

DISTANCE & CONFIGURATION: 4.7-mile loop

HIKING TIME: 2–3 hours

HIGHLIGHTS: Bog, nature trail guide, abandoned farmstead, passport trail

ELEVATION: 1,370' at trailhead; 1,880' at highest point along loop

ACCESS: Open 24/7; no fees or permits required

MAPS: Finger Lakes Trail Conference: Sheet B3; DEC Urbana State Forest map:
dec.ny.gov/lands/37442.html

FACILITIES: None

WHEELCHAIR ACCESS: No

COMMENTS: Based on the usual trail rating system, a five-star rating in the "Children" category might seem to indicate that you can bring kids in strollers. This is certainly not the case here, as there is a very steep climb that will be challenging for many children and impossible for strollers. Why the five stars then? Unique to this trip is the *Nature Trail Guide* (described later) provided along the trail, which I think will prove an excellent resource for educating children and teaching them about nature. Of course, to appreciate this, children should be capable of the steep climb and the trip length of 4.7 miles, but for the budding naturalist—young or old—I think this trail rates five stars.

CONTACTS: NYSDEC Region 8 Headquarters, 607-776-2165, **dec.ny.gov/lands/37442.html**

Overview

Though the initial climb may prove challenging, once you reach the top of the plateau, the trail is mostly level hiking. In each of the trail registers, an excellent *Nature Trail Guide* introduces hikers to many of the natural and historic features found along the trail. It's an excellent companion for exploring the upland bog, and I highly recommend you bring one along (see details below).

Route Details

From the small pulloff on the north side of Bean Station Road, head across the street to the orange-painted bridge that crosses the drainage ditch. A green street sign labeled "Cemetery" also marks the bridge and trailhead. Head south past the white sign with red-painted lettering; the sign indicates that the private property you are now traversing is made accessible to hikers and skiers only. For approximately the first 0.5 mile you will be on private property, so please respect property rights and stay on the designated trail. The trail quickly begins its ascent, and you soon pass through an open lawn beside a cemetery. The trail continues straight, marked with orange paints, past the Covell Cemetery, and heads into the forest. The ascent is along a broad forest road and is fairly brisk—more than 400 feet of elevation gain in less than 0.6 mile.

About 0.25 mile in, you pass a log trail shelter on your left. This is the Evangeline trail shelter, which is privately owned but available for public use on a first-come, first-serve basis. If the generosity of a private landowner providing a shelter for hikers strikes you as unique, consider that this shelter is actually in its second generation. The original shelter, built by volunteers and AmeriCorps, was an instant success but unfortunately was burned down by some irresponsible local kids. Many would expect such an event to sour private landowners from continuing their generous sharing; instead, this property owner had the shelter rebuilt, bigger and better than before, and it is still available without restriction.

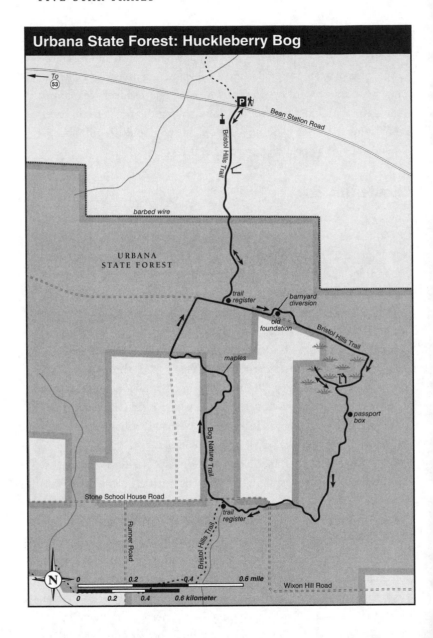

Urbana State Forest: Huckleberry Bog

To 53

Bean Station Road

Bristol Hills Trail

barbed wire

URBANA
STATE FOREST

trail register

barnyard diversion

old foundation

Bristol Hills Trail

maples

Bog Nature Trail

passport box

Stone School House Road

Runner Road

Bristol Hills Trail

trail register

Wixon Hill Road

N

0   0.2   0.4   0.6 mile

0   0.2   0.4   0.6 kilometer

At 0.4 mile, you reach some barbed wire along the trail. This marks the end of the private-property section of the trail, and as you pass through an open section in the fence, you will see warning signs indicating just that. Past the fence, the trail begins to level off, but you don't truly reach the top of the climb until you arrive at the north Huckleberry Bog Trail register and junction with a light blue–marked trail, 0.4 mile ahead (0.8 mile overall).

Now if you eschew trail registers, you are going to miss out on a very special treat. Inside are laminated copies of the *Huckleberry Bog Nature Trail Guide*. The 44-page guide is the latest edition of an evolving collaboration between trail stewards, naturalists, students, and the Finger Lakes Trail Conference (FLTC). Hikers are welcome to *borrow* the guide while they are on the trail but must return the guides to the register in which they were found. The guides are truly excellent and provide in-depth information about specific features along the trail. Plant identification drawings and descriptions are also included within the guides and are helpful while exploring this upland bog. Again *please don't remove* these guides from the trail. If you enjoy the information or wish to read more later, then download the guide for *free* at **fltconference.org/trail/go-hiking/special-places /huckleberry-bog.**

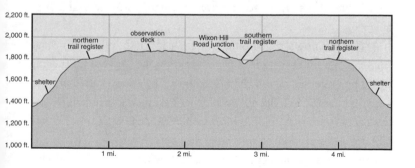

To begin the loop, continue straight, following orange blazes. Very quickly you intersect an old road. Turn left onto the road, and shortly after you will pass the first stop (#1) described within the *Nature Trail Guide*, a white disc with a green-painted number one affixed to an apple tree. I won't describe each stop along the trail (when I visited, there were 46 stops) because the guide provides more than sufficient information. Rather, I wanted to point out what to look for as you explore the trail and guide.

Continue easterly along the road about 0.25 mile to where the trail turns sharply left into the forest near an old foundation. Several stops are found here at the old Depew homestead, and the "barnyard detour" quickly leads back to the forest road you were previously following. Back along the road, you continue another 0.25 mile east, to a sharp right turn along the trail near stop number 12. You are now 1.3 miles from the start; as you head south keep an eye out for the bog to appear on your right.

At approximately 1.5 miles, you reach the observation deck at the eastern edge of the bog. A very short distance farther you intersect a fork in the trail; to the right is a side trip, marked in blue, that takes you 0.1 mile farther into the bog, while to the left is the continuation of the orange trail. Unfortunately, I visited the bog on a cold drizzling day when wildlife activity was low, but should you proceed quietly here, I imagine that you might catch sight of some interesting wildlife. This short dead-end trail concludes abruptly near a large fallen log.

To continue along the main trail, head south following orange paints, either by bearing left if you forgo the side trip or by turning right upon returning from the side trip. Pass by a large vernal pool on your right (stop 23) followed by a Finger Lakes passport mailbox (see the Connecticut Hill Wildlife Management Area: Bob Cameron Loop, 189, for a description of this program). Soon after, you pass by the "hugging trees," a large hemlock and oak whose trunks intertwine near their bases, providing a most unusual sight on your right, at 1.9 miles from the start. The trail continues less than 0.5 mile south before bearing to the west. Aside from the various nature guide stops, the trail is relatively uneventful until just shy of 2.5 miles, where you cross Wixon Hill Road. Little more than a worn and rutted logging road, Wixon Hill Road bisects the trail and leads down to some open water on your right. However, this open water lies on private property that is essentially encircled by Urbana State Forest. Continue straight across the road, past stop number 44, and rock-hop across a small stream. After crossing this tributary stream of Keuka Lake, you pass the final nature stop, number 46, and soon reach the south Huckleberry Bog Trail register. The register also marks a trail intersection; to the left is the continuation of the Bristol Hills Trail, marked in orange, while to the right is the light blue–marked return leg of our loop. If you don't plan to continue the loop, leave your nature guide here. However, if you are continuing along the loop, then bring your guide back to the north register for other loop hikers to enjoy.

To continue the loop, turn right and head north. The trail reconnects and briefly climbs along Wixon Hill Road. Keep an eye out for the double blue paints that mark the turnoff, just past a gnarly old pine on your right. Continue heading north up a short climb to what is the highest elevation along the trail, between 1,870 and 1,880 feet. The trail traverses a narrow strip of public land between two privately owned properties whose property lines and related signs often neighbor the trail. The path is clearly marked and you are unlikely to go astray.

At approximately 3 miles, the trail turns to the right (east) and heads into a stand of beech trees. Shortly after this turn, the trail resumes its northerly course for about 0.25 mile, where it bends to the west. You will follow along an old row of tall maples with cobbles strewn about their bases, typical of an old field edge or property boundary. Shy of 3.5 miles, you intersect an old logging road coming in from your left, or the south. Turn right onto this old road and head northeast back to the northern trail register. Return your nature guide to the trail register and head back along the orange trail downhill to your car on Bean Station Road, another 0.8 mile ahead. The total trip length is 4.7 miles.

Directions

From points north: From the intersection of NY 14A and NY 54A in Penn Yan, head west along NY 54A South/West Lake Road. After 7.5 miles, turn left to remain on NY 54A South/West Lake Road. Turn right on Gibson Hill Road after 7.1 miles. Turn left onto Middle Road at 0.2 mile. Follow Middle Road for 1.8 miles and bear right onto Shuart Road. Cross CR 76/South Pulteney Road and continue onto CR 77. Turn left on Depew Road, at 1.7 miles. Take a sharp left onto Bean Station Road at 0.3 mile. Continue 1.1 miles on Bean Station Road to the parking area on the right.

From points south: From I-86, take Exit 37 (NY 53, Kanona/Prattsburg). Turn right onto NY 53 North and follow it for 8.8 miles. Turn right onto Bean Station Road. Follow Bean Station Road 2.6 miles and look for the small pulloff on the left side of the road.

Appendix A:
Further Reading

Geology

Allman, Warren D. and Robert M. Ross. *Ithaca is Gorges: A Guide to the Geology of the Ithaca Area*. Ithaca, NY: The Paleontological Research Institute, 2011.

Ansley, J. E. *The Teacher-Friendly Guide to the Geology of the Northeastern U.S.* Ithaca, NY: The Paleontological Research Institution, 2000. geology.teacherfriendlyguide.org

Van Diver, Bradford B. *Roadside Geology of New York*. Missoula, MT: Mountain Press Publishing Company, 1985.

Von Engeln, O. D. *The Finger Lakes Region*. Ithaca, NY: Cornell University Press, 1995.

Waterfalls

Brown, Scott E. *New York Waterfalls: A Guide for Hikers & Photographers*. Mechanicsburg, PA: Stackpole Books, 2010.

Ensminger, Scott A. with David J. Schryver and Edward M. Smathers. *Waterfalls of New York State*. Buffalo, NY: Firefly Books, 2012.

Freeman, Rich and Sue Freeman. *200 Waterfalls in Central & Western New York*. Englewood, FL: Footprint Press, 2010.

Camping

Starmer, Aaron with Cate Starmer and Timothy Starmer. *Best Tent Camping: New York State*. Birmingham, AL: Menasha Ridge Press, 2013.

Appendix B:
Map Resources

The Finger Lakes Trail Conference (FLTC) is the best source of maps for the region. Maps are available as print and digital editions and are very reasonably priced; part of the proceeds go to further enhancing the trails in the region.

Finger Lakes Trail Conference, 585-658-9320, **fltconference.org**

Maps for land trust properties, along with biographical information regarding each property, are online.

Finger Lakes Land Trust, 607-275-9487, **fllt.org**

State park maps are often online, but the print versions at entrance booths and park offices are often better.

NYS Office of Parks, Recreation and Historic Preservation, nysparks.com

Department of Environmental Conservation maps are online but are the least informative. However, occasionally they are the only option besides this book. Look for an FLTC map that covers the same area whenever possible.

New York State Department of Environmental Conservation, 518-473-9518, **dec.ny.gov/outdoor/351.html**

Appendix C: Trail Clubs

ADIRONDACK MOUNTAIN CLUB, ONONDAGA CHAPTER: adk-on.org

CAYUGA TRAILS CLUB: cayugatrailsclub.org

FINGER LAKES TRAIL CONFERENCE:
585-658-9320, **fltconference.org**

NORTH COUNTRY TRAIL ASSOCIATION, CENTRAL NEW YORK CHAPTER:
nctacnychapter.org

SYRACUSE AREA OUTDOOR ADVENTURE CLUB:
meetup.com/adventurers-103

Index

About the Author

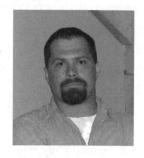

TIM STARMER HAS ALWAYS BEEN AN OUT-DOORS ENTHUSIAST. He spent most of his childhood seeking out remote, wild areas whenever possible. Throughout his life the Adirondacks and its vast wilderness have been one of Starmer's favorite destinations for hiking and backpacking trips. During a brief hiatus from Brown University in 1997, he spent six weeks driving across the United States, camping the entire way. Along the way he explored many of the West's national and state parks, including Canyonlands, Yellowstone, Arches, Bryce Canyon—he even braved pitching a tent among the mosquito swarms in Badlands National Park. At the trip's conclusion, he headed to Australia, where he backpacked for a few months exploring the eastern outback, the Great Barrier Reef, and the caves of Tasmania, as well as traversing the Tasmanian Wilderness World Heritage Area along the Overland Track. In 2006 Starmer was thrilled to have the opportunity to explore numerous wilderness gems across New York when he coauthored *Best Tent Camping: New York State*. His second book, *Five-Star Trails in the Adirondacks*, was published in 2010 and features some of the best trails in the Adirondack Park. Starmer owns and operates New Heritage Woodworking, a construction company that specializes in designing and building timber frames in Upstate New York.

DEAR CUSTOMERS AND FRIENDS,

SUPPORTING YOUR INTEREST IN OUTDOOR ADVENTURE, travel, and an active lifestyle is central to our operations, from the authors we choose to the locations we detail to the way we design our books. Menasha Ridge Press was incorporated in 1982 by a group of veteran outdoorsmen and professional outfitters. For many years now, we've specialized in creating books that benefit the outdoors enthusiast.

Almost immediately, Menasha Ridge Press earned a reputation for revolutionizing outdoors- and travel-guidebook publishing. For such activities as canoeing, kayaking, hiking, backpacking, and mountain biking, we established new standards of quality that transformed the whole genre, resulting in outdoor-recreation guides of great sophistication and solid content. Menasha Ridge continues to be outdoor publishing's greatest innovator.

The folks at Menasha Ridge Press are as at home on a whitewater river or mountain trail as they are editing a manuscript. The books we build for you are the best they can be, because we're responding to your needs. Plus, we use and depend on them ourselves.

We look forward to seeing you on the river or the trail. If you'd like to contact us directly, join in at trekalong.com or visit us at menasharidge .com. We thank you for your interest in our books and the natural world around us all.

SAFE TRAVELS,

Bob Sehlinger

BOB SEHLINGER
PUBLISHER